The Magic Therapy of Colours

A.R. Hari

Pustak Mahal®
Delhi • Mumbai • Bangalore
Patna • Hyderabad

Publishers
Pustak Mahal, Delhi-110006

Sales Centres
- 6686, Khari Baoli, Delhi-110006, *Ph:* 23944314, 23911979
- 10-B, Netaji Subhash Marg, Daryaganj, New Delhi-110002
  Ph: 23268292, 23268293, 23279900 • *Fax:* 011-23280567

Administrative Office
J-3/16 (Opp. Happy School), Daryaganj, New Delhi-110002
Ph: 23276539, 23272783, 23272784 • *Fax:* 011-23260518
E-mail: info@pustakmahal.com • *Website:* www.pustakmahal.com

Branch Offices

BANGALORE: 22/2, Mission Road (Shama Rao's Compound), Bangalore-560027, *Ph:* 2234025 • *Fax:* 080-2240209
E-mail: pmblr@sancharnet.in • pustak@sancharnet.in

MUMBAI: 23-25, Zaoba Wadi (Opp. VIP Showroom), Thakurdwar, Mumbai-400002, *Ph:* 22010941 • *Fax:* 022-22053387
E-mail: rapidex@bom5.vsnl.net.in

PATNA: Khemka House, 1st Floor (Opp. Women's Hospital), Ashok Rajpath, Patna-800004, *Telefax:* 0612-2673644
E-mail: rapidexptn@rediffmail.com

HYDERABAD: 5-1-707/1, Brij Bhawan, Bank Street, Koti, Hyderabad-500095, *Ph:* 24737530 • *Fax:* 040-24737290
E-mail: pustakmahal-hyd@indiatimes.com

ISBN 81-223-0833-3

Edition : June 2003

Printed at: Unique Color Carton, New Delhi 110064

Preface

Colour therapy has been in vogue since ancient times. Hindus have always considered different colours as manifestations of the Supreme Lord.

The following lines succinctly outline the relationship between colours and God:

Evamesha mahadevo deva deva pitaamaha
Karomi niyathakalam kalatma eiswari thanuhu
Vishwame rasamayo vipra sarvaloka pradeepakaha
Thesham shreshta punanha
Saptarasamayo tanayee namaha

–Kurma Purana

The Lord is supreme and is the God of gods. He controls time and time rests in Him. He illumines the world with His brilliant hues. Of these, seven are most important and I bow to them.

It is quite clear that much before Western scientists proved through the prism spectrum that white light was made up of seven colours, ancient Indian sages were well aware of this fact.

From the early stages of human evolution colour has aroused the interest of man. This is quite natural as nature is filled with colour. Everywhere we look around us, greenery is predominant in nature.

There are other rich colours in nature, too.

The sky is blue, but takes on breathtaking hues when the sun's rays play with the clouds during sunset. At such times, one can see red as well as violet, which lights up the entire sky. The rainbow is another beautiful phenomenon where all the seven colours in the spectrum stand out brilliantly across the sky.

Flowers are another example of nature's bounty seen in innumerable colours. Almost all permutations and combinations that man can ever think of already exist in nature. The colour preference of nature indicates that nature is fully aware of the beauty associated with colours and utilises it to the maximum to make God's creations appear even more spectacular.

Apart from flowers, beautiful birds with kaleidoscopic shades inhabit various parts of the globe, contributing their mite to making the world more beautiful. It is therefore not surprising that man noticed colours and has enjoyed their beauty since ancient times.

This interest in colour must have goaded the ancients to examine the impact of colour upon the mind and body. There is little doubt that given its past heritage, India is the birthplace of chromo-therapy. However, the scattering of light into various colours through the use of prisms, the advent of coloured glasses and other advances by the West helped colour therapy take giant strides.

Colour therapy has come of age and is today recognised as a respectable, holistic method of treatment. Research on colour therapy is being conducted around the world. The current findings are sufficient to justify the application of colour therapy in many disorders to which the human body is prone. Significantly, in the hands of a trained practitioner, colour therapy is safe, harmless and relatively inexpensive in India.

This book aims to enlighten the readers on the latest research and breakthroughs in this field. The book is therefore unique as it updates you on the latest research findings.

The application of colour in modern times is more important than ever before. Earlier generations had the good fortune of being exposed to nature, when they could enjoy its beauty and receive vibrations from various colours. This helped them have a cheerful mind and healthy body.

Today, this is no longer true. Modern man spends most of his life cooped up either in a drawing hall, in the office or in an automobile. He rarely looks up at the sky or has any time to enjoy nature. Thanks to the odd hours they keep, some people even spend a few months without being exposed to the sun.

In such a situation, the body is the casualty, missing out on the invigorating colour vibrations present in nature. There is no doubt that the high energy levels and the good health enjoyed by the ancients was partly due to the fact that they allowed all colours in nature to work on them by staying out in the open during the day. The body is blessed with inherent intelligence and knows what colour is required to repair which organ. As all colours are freely available in nature, the vibrations were absorbed effortlessly, resulting in vibrant health for everyone.

This luxury is largely denied to us today. To some extent, having the right healthy colours in the interiors of our houses and offices can rectify this shortcoming.

The Magic Therapy of Colours deals with the history of colour therapy, the modern methods of utilising colour therapy and the areas where it is beneficial. The book will therefore be a valuable guide for those who wish to benefit from colour and colour therapy.

–A.R. Hari

Contents

The History of Colour Therapy 9

The Basic Principles 16

Application of Colour in Modern Medicine 18

How Colours Affect Us 22

Colours and Chakras in the Human Body 25

Methods of Administering Colour Therapy 30

Spot Application of Colour Therapy 32

Sources of Colour 83

Colour Breathing Techniques 90

Colour Combination Treatment 94

Colour Therapy Through Chakras 100

Acupuncture and LED Light Colour Therapy 103

Energy Colour Healing 106

Octagonal Colour Pyramid 110

Use of Colour Pyramid Water 112

Pyramid Healing Through Chakras 114

Colour Crystal Cards 116

The History of Colour Therapy

White colour consists of seven different colours and can be split into its constituent colours by using a prism.

The seven colours that make up white light are:

- Violet
- Indigo
- Blue
- Green
- Yellow
- Orange
- Red

The ancient Egyptians believed that their God Thoth was the one who developed healing with colour. The ancient Greeks were also using colour to treat various diseases. They had come to the conclusion that the human body contained various coloured fluids – like bile (yellow), blood (red), phlegm (white) and so on. They thought that these were connected with the functioning of the spleen, the heart, the liver and the brain and believed that good health resulted when these humours were present in the right proportion.

In an effort to cure a person of his illness, they used coloured garments, coloured plasters and the like.

In the first century AD, Aurelius Cornelius developed the doctrine of medicine established by Hippocrates where he mentioned the use of coloured ointments and coloured flowers in medicine.

Arab philosopher and physician Ibn Sina (AD 980–AD 1037) expounded the theory of colour healing in his book *Canon of Medicine* and was the first to indicate that red colour improved the quality of blood, white colour purified it and yellow colour reduced pain and inflammation. Known as Avicenna in the West, Ibn Sina recommended potions of yellow flowers to cure bile disorders and red flowers to cure blood disorders. He also gave contraindications for colour usage, wherein he advocated a ban on red colour in case of haemorrhoids.

Theophratus Bombastus von Hohenheim – a renowned healer, popularly known as Dr Paracelsus (1493–1541) – openly confessed he had gained his knowledge about the laws and practices of colour medicine from conversations with witches. In medieval times, witches were strongly dealt with by the Church and ordinary citizens were forbidden from having contact with them. Dr Paracelsus regarded light and colour as very essential to maintaining good health and used them therapeutically by exposing herbs and preparing elixirs to treat various conditions. He was successful in treating a variety of ailments by his methods and people from all over Europe visited him seeking cures.

During the Middle Ages, colour therapies lost credibility with the rapid strides made by science, which placed colour therapists in a difficult situation since they could not satisfactorily explain how colours achieved healing.

Rationalism, reason and appraisal became critical factors for the acceptance of a finding. Only what was certain and evident was accepted and whatever was doubtful was rejected. Gradually, the emphasis changed from the spiritual to the material. Medicine concentrated on the physical body, entirely ignoring the mind and spirit. Advances in surgery, the discovery of powerful antibiotics such as penicillin and their phenomenal success simply pushed healing systems like colour therapy into the distant background.

All the same, research in colour healing continued to survive in odd pockets, although it had lost much of its significance and no longer attracted public interest.

In 1876, the Frenchman Augustus Pleasanton published a book, *Blue and Sunlight*, in which he claimed that grapes grown in greenhouses with alternate blue and transparent panes of glasses increased the yield. He also claimed that blue light could treat disease and pain in humans. He credited colours with other attributes such as increased fertility in animals and physical maturation.

Another distinguished physician of the times, Dr Seth Pancoast published *Blue and Red Lights* in 1877, wherein he endorsed the findings of Augustus Pleasanton. In 1896, the book *Principles of Light and Colour*, published by Edwin Babbitt, became one of the most popular books of the time. Babbitt identified various colours with the organs and systems that they primarily affect. For example, red colour was identified as a stimulant of blood and yellow and orange as nerve stimulants. Blue and violet were identified as soothing and anti-inflammatory. Based on these qualities, red colour was recommended in chronic rheumatism, yellow as a laxative, blue in inflammatory conditions, etc.

He developed various devices and named them 'Thermolume', which used colour glasses to produce coloured light, and 'chromo-disk', which centred a coloured light beam on desired parts of the human body. Babbitt also developed the method of exposing water to various coloured lights and claimed that consumption of this water could cure various diseases. This method of treatment is still in vogue.

Following Babbitt's discovery, quite a few people began practising this system of healing, calling themselves chromopaths. At the end of the nineteenth century, red light was used to prevent scars in cases of smallpox and patients with tuberculosis were treated with sunlight, to cite just two examples.

The medical fraternity was not impressed and by and large ignored the therapy. In the early twentieth century, the Austrian social philosopher Rudolph Steiner (1861–1925) suggested that there is a strong connection between colour, form, shape and sound.

In other words, certain combinations of colour can have regenerative or destructive effects. Theo Gimbel, who founded the Hygeia College of Colour Therapy in Britain, corroborated Steiner's work. Several distinguished personalities such as Max Luscher, Professor of Psychology at Basle University, joined Gimbel to promote colour therapy.

Luscher's theory was that the preference of colour by a person indicated the imbalance and could be used both for psychological and physical diagnosis. Luscher opined that early man had known only two colours with which he was familiar, viz., day and night. These two colours controlled all activities in the human body, the functioning of various organs, sleeping and waking.

In other words, the human organism has the control points in nature that alternates between day and night. Day stands for putting the body into activity and motion, while night returns the body to a state of rest through sleep, which relaxes and rejuvenates all parts of the body.

Luscher related bright yellow (an artificial colour) to 'day' and dark blue (another artificial colour) to 'night'. He stated that metabolic secretion from various glands could all be controlled by application of these two colours. The only factor to determine was whether the organ needed stimulation or rest.

For instance, if stimulation was required for organs in the digestive system, then it was concluded that they needed the day colour to energise them. If the organ was overworked, then deep sleep and rest were required to nurse it back to health and, in this case, night colours were required to rest and relax the system. If a person suffered from lack of sleep, night colours were obviously required to get restful sleep.

In 1940, Russian scientist S.V. Krakov proved that red stimulates the sympathetic part of the dynamic nervous system, while blue stimulates the parasympathetic part. These findings were later confirmed through an independent study conducted by Robert Gerard in 1958.

Gerard went deeper and came to the conclusion that anxiety was directly related to red while tranquillity was related to blue. He conclusively proved that exposing blood pressure patients to soothing blue lights could control blood pressure. According to Gerard, patients suffering from anxiety-neurosis (a nervous disorder that keeps a person on edge) could be effectively calmed by the application of blue colour, which released body tranquillisers and helped the patient overcome anxiety.

Remarking on the effects of various colours on human physiology, Dr Harry Wolfforth showed that blood pressure, pulse and respiration sharply go up under yellow light, moderately increase under orange light and minimally under red. They decrease very much in black, moderately under blue and minimally under green. Experiments carried out on rats showed that when kept in red colour, their appetite and growth rate increased.

It was in the 1960s when modern medicine finally accepted that neo-natal jaundice (a viral condition found in two-thirds of premature babies) could be successfully treated with blue light.

Modern research indicates that every cell in the body emits light and can be stimulated by external application of colour. Based on this theory, colour acupuncture points have been picked up and instead of inserting needles, only a beam of light is centred at that point. This has been found to be a quick and effective means of healing.

The oriental system is however based on healing the chakras, which in turn sets right the defect in the organs.

Today, orthodox medicine uses colour therapy by exposing children with neo-natal jaundice to blue colour, which is believed to boost the immune system. Colour therapy has brought substantial relief in cases of insomnia, anxiety, asthma, behavioural and learning disorders and can aid faster recoveries from surgeries.

Currently, the International Association of Colour Therapy Practitioners, located in London, has hundreds of members from all over the world. Every member who wants to practise colour therapy is required to register himself with this organisation before treating patients.

Some questions put to the Ascended Master Maha Chohan by a viewer have elicited interesting answers. Ascended Masters are enlightened spiritual beings who once lived on earth. They completed their mission and ascended back to their divine source. They are believed to continue to live in their etheric bodies. Masters give insights on secret knowledge to chosen ones when they are in a deep meditative state. The Maha Chohan sect is located in Sri Lanka. It is believed that there are eight such masters who have ascended and guided seekers in their spiritual quest.

The following question-and-answer session between an ardent devotee and Ascended Master Maha Chohan will be enlightening to those interested in colour therapy:

Do you think a colour-filled environment is necessary in a children's hospital?

Colour is the next phase of high vibration healing. Children can be highly sensitised to the healing properties of colour, especially at this time of raised vibration. The way of viewing colour is now old and non-functional. Interior design schools are way behind what the human is in need of.

Whether adult, child or animal, a living being senses colour on many levels. In fact, the body's intelligence perceives colour in multi-dimensions. It is not about making a room pretty. It sets a vibration tone (sound) that affects the sensory system of a human form. There have been many human studies on the psychology of colour and how it affects the mind. This is not entirely correct. It affects all of the body's sensors at different body levels – causal body, astral body and the physical body.

The physical body sends out feelers to experience the sensation. The colour is just energy. Energy is taken in various ways and intention can play a part in this process. Ancient studies knew this. Because humans are always seeking gratification outside themselves, they see colour as a form of unimportant decoration to match a theme. In fact the theme they are so attached to is a past or future life they have experienced/will experience.

People who are partial to oriental, ethnic items or any culture, and their colorations, recall through sensory perception that feeling of before. Colour is a fascinating area to concentrate on. It is in fact going to be the next way you will heal. Light is also part of that process. It is possible to heal people by bathing them in a specific colour, whether it is a room or clothes.

On a very deep level of DNA, it affects the chromosomes and cellular complement. I am sorry you will not find this in books yet. Many are starting to become awakened to what colour will do.

Every colour is said to have a specific emotional effect on people. If a children's ward or room is painted in a specific colour scheme, which is chosen to have a therapeutic effect on the patients, how effectively do you think it would work?
If a sick child who's constantly in pain spent most of the time in a dominantly blue room, it is said by some therapists to have a 'soothing and calming effect'.

Do you think that in general everybody reacts the same way to colours? Or do you think it depends on the individual and things such as culture, mental state etc?
Reaction to colour on an individual basis depends on how clear a vibration they are operating at. Reaction is quite subliminal on an unconscious level. I suggest you experiment with colour and test people's reactions.

In the above answer, Maha Chohan indicates that the reaction of an individual to colour is somewhat unique and every person need not react in the same way. For example, in an atmosphere filled with blue colour, healing does take place. But the extent of healing varies from person to person. There could be cases where the colour has no effect on the individual at all. If an organism lacks sensitivity to colour vibrations, then it may not be in a position to draw energy from it.

The Basic Principles

Colour therapists believe that the hypothalamus in the human body controls the pituitary gland and as the former is influenced by light, it acts on the pituitary gland, which in turn controls all the other glands like the pineal, thyroid, thymus, adrenalin, pancreas, ovaries, etc.

The pineal gland responds to light and produces melatonin, which is involved in maintaining the metabolic rhythm. Mystics believe that the pineal gland is linked to the *Sahasrara Chakra* on top of the head.

Colour therapy uses the sensitivity of a person to colour to identify and correct any imbalance in the body's internal energy patterns that may be the cause of emotional or physical ill health.

According to colour therapists, every organ system has its own vibration energy and disease can occur when this energy is short. By applying the same colour, which has the same vibration energy, the disease can be overcome. Blue, yellow and red are identified as principal colours.

Modern physics has established that every colour has a certain frequency wavelength and energy associated with it. Therefore, the colour we absorb affects our nervous and endocrine system, and eventually the release of hormones and other organic substances within the human body. Hence, the disease indicates that there is improper utilisation of colour and a cure lies in the application of the right colour frequency.

Colour therapy can be administered in various ways. In earlier times, gems were used for colour therapy. Presently, several methods for administering colour therapy are practised worldwide.

Breathing exercises conducted when the eyes are looking at a specific colour are believed to help the body absorb colour vibrations.

Crystals are available in various colours. When light passes through them, the corresponding colour light is obtained, which can be used for therapeutic purposes.

Coloured garments are another way of administering colour therapy. By covering an organ that needs vibration with a coloured cloth, the desired energy can be passed on to a person.

Coloured water – also termed 'solarised' water – is another popular method wherein coloured bottles containing water are exposed to sunlight for some time.

Another modern method is through coloured lights using electrical bulbs, whereby the patient is exposed to the required colour.

Monochromatic light is another form of colour therapy, which combines acupuncture to pass on colour vibrations.

All these methods are discussed in detail in the subsequent chapters.

Application of Colour in Modern Medicine

Modern research has shown that colour indeed has an effect on our mood and health. Lack of natural daylight impairs our mood and if one is exposed to artificial light for most part of the day, the quality of life will be greatly affected.

Ordinary, cool, white fluorescent lamps have an unbalanced spectral distribution and distort other colours, straining the eye and the system. Now, full-spectrum fluorescent lamps are manufactured abroad, which give light in the same colour temperature as that of sunlight. This exactly matches the bright, white sunlight one sees during the day. Exposure to this light has reportedly brought relief in various types of glandular disorders, insomnia, fatigue, depression, Alzheimer's disease and other ailments.

Blue light is found to be effective in the treatment of rheumatoid arthritis, a joint disorder that has so far remained elusive to cures by modern medicine. There is no proven medicine except a recommended regimen of vitamins, painkillers and physiotherapy to check the progress of this disease.

Further, once the disease sets in, the progress cannot be stopped, but only slowed down. Painkillers are not without side effects and after a period of time, immunity develops, with the result that stronger and higher dosages are required for the same effect. The disease continues its relentless march towards total incapacitation and leads to a condition where the patient will not be able to carry out his daily activities.

According to Dr SF McDonald, blue light brought significant relief from pain in such cases. Blue light is also used in the treatment of non-malignant tumours and cancers.

At the annual conference of the American Association for Advancement of Science in 1990, scientists reported that blue light could be used successfully to treat psychological problems and other diseases. Migraines, headaches and certain forms of cancer respond positively to red light.

Modern medicine is slowly looking at colour as another therapeutic tool. Photodynamic therapy is an offshoot of such experiments, wherein certain photosensitive chemicals are injected into the body. They only accumulate in cancer cells, identify such cells and destroy these when they are activated by red light.

More than 3,000 people have responded favourably to treatment by this technique.

The colour pink has been found to be a tranquilliser and has a calming effect within minutes of exposure. Hostile and aggressive people can be turned into more agreeable types and it is almost an acknowledged fact that in pink surroundings, people cannot be aggressive, even if they want to, because the colour saps their energy.

By contrast, yellow light encourages violence. In fact, an increase in violence all over the world is attributed to some extent to the wide use of sodium vapour lamps, which emits a yellow hue.

Similarly, people suffering from the learning disorder, dyslexia, respond favourably to colour therapy. Doctors have found that having these children put on tinted glasses could make them see letters properly. The British Medical Research Council has confirmed this in 1993. In Britain, an Intuitive Colour Meter is developed to select the right colour glass for people suffering from dyslexia.

The paranormal effects of colour have also become a subject of study. Scientists are hard put to explain phenomenon like 'eyeless sight' of persons who are totally blind, yet able to recognise colours.

A new term, Dermo-optic Vision, has been coined to explain this phenomenon according to which even skin on the human body is capable of responding to colour stimulations. It is believed that almost one in six persons has this unique ability of identifying colours even when blindfolded, although most are not aware of this faculty.

Similarly, such subjects were able to identify colours correctly when coloured objects covered with various materials like brass, copper and aluminium plates were given to them.

It is believed that the pineal gland may be behind the manifestation of this unique ability. The pineal gland produces two hormones called melatonin and serotonin. Melatonin is an important chemical which helps animals respond to light and synchronises their body reactions to the daily cycle.

Serotonin is another very important chemical of the brain that is responsible for behavioural patterns. During a span of 24 hours, serotonin is produced during the day and melatonin during the night. Depression appears to be linked with melatonin levels. Naturally, sunlight alleviates this problem by controlling melatonin release.

Specific colours appear to affect specific diseases. Eruptive diseases respond better in a room with red windows. Similarly, people under stress or depression recover rapidly when they are placed in rooms with red light. Pain is relieved when patients are subjected to flashing and coloured lights.

Scientists believe that the brain itself is colour sensitive and responds to different frequencies of various colours. Using blue colour, for example, can effectively cure sleep problems. Violet light induces relaxation, reduces stress and chronic pain.

Research on colour therapy is continuing in various parts of the world and several university hospitals abroad have allowed their post-graduate degree students to conduct their thesis research on colour therapy projects. A section of modern medical practitioners believes that colour therapy has a bright future.

Dr Harry Riley of the United States documented that profound physiological and psychological changes were induced in patients when the colour of light entering their eyes was changed. These experiments have made the scientific community look more closely at the spectrum itself.

According to current research, the spectrum is believed to contain eight colours (instead of seven as believed earlier): Red, Orange, Yellow, Green, Turquoise, Blue, Violet and Magenta. Modern colour therapists put all these colours to use in curing various ailments.

ooo

How Colours Affect Us

Colour can affect us on the physical, emotional, mental and spiritual planes, since man exists in all the four states simultaneously. An illness can be attributed to a disturbance in any one plane, although the effect may be seen in other planes as well.

For example, if a person has an upset stomach, it may be due to a physical disorder but he will also be emotionally disturbed and mentally tense. The same effect can be perceived when a person is emotionally upset, as it can again cause disturbance at the physical level, resulting in loss of appetite or indigestion.

In the first case, the cause is physical and, therefore, colour therapy is to be administered at the physical level. If the cause is emotional, the treatment is to be administered at the emotional level. This factor is very important because the choice of colour in each case is different.

Let us see how colours affect us on the physical, emotional, mental and spiritual planes.

On the physical plane

- Green and light blue make us restful.
- Orange is revitalising.
- Red stimulates.

On the emotional plane

- Sky blue and turquoise are restful.
- Peach is revitalising.
- Orange is stimulating.

On the mental plane

- Indigo is restful.
- Emerald green revitalises.

- Yellow stimulates.

On the spiritual plane

- Blue is restful.
- Gold revitalises.
- Violet and purple stimulate.

On the physical level, green and light blue relax, orange has a revitalising effect and red stimulates. These colours can affect us on the emotional, mental and spiritual levels also.

Therefore, the colour combinations for restful sleep are sky blue or turquoise, whereas for revitalising emotions one has to use peach. Emotions are also stimulated by the colour orange. At the mental level, indigo induces restfulness, whereas emerald green revitalises. Yellow stimulates mental acumen.

If one is looking for spiritual progress, then purple appears restful, whereas the colour gold revitalises. Violet acts as a stimulator. Those engaged in meditation should use violet in the meditation room.

It is important to recognise at what level the therapy is required, whether physical, mental or emotional. If the therapy is required at the physical level, then it has to be decided whether it is required to stimulate or to shake off lethargy and revitalise one to counter the effects of excessive strain.

Similarly, on the emotional level, if the therapy is to be administered and a person is emotionally not responsive, he needs the colour orange to revitalise him.

However, if emotions have drained the person, he needs a more restful colour like peach to revitalise him. On the mental level, if the person is mentally tired by excess work, one should use indigo to induce restfulness.

A person who feels drained of ideas can be revitalised with emerald, whereas indigo should be selected if a person has a mind clouded with thoughts. If the person has a disinterested outlook towards life, the colour yellow can change his attitude.

On the spiritual level, one has to be very relaxed to secure any result and, therefore, blue is recommended. If meditation practices are taxing, the colour gold is recommended to revitalise oneself. Again, during meditation there can be frustration and lack of interest if the desired progress is not achieved. In such cases, one should use violet.

The above information is very important while selecting a colour for therapeutic purposes. The job of the colour therapist is indeed complex, as he has to identify the seat of the disease and determine whether the cause is physical, emotional, mental or spiritual. Any mistake here will result in a wasted effort.

Therefore, the role of a colour therapist in curing ailments is becoming more important as the popularity of this system grows.

OOO

Colours and Chakras in the Human Body

Understanding the concept of the chakras is pivotal to understanding the universe. *Chakra* is a Sanskrit word which means *wheel* and the credit for finding this path to ultimate knowledge goes to Hinduism. The entire concept of Yoga revolves around chakras.

Yoga is probably the only system that uses the physical body as a vehicle to reach the highest stage of spiritual consciousness. Yoga believes it is the spinal column that holds the secret path to knowledge and liberation. This is supposed to contain three *nadis* or channels called *Ida, Pingala* and *Sushumna.*

In an ordinary human being, the *Sushumna* is closed and only the *Ida* and *Pingala,* which correspond to the left and right nostrils, operate. The spinal cord has the following chakras or wheels situated over its length.

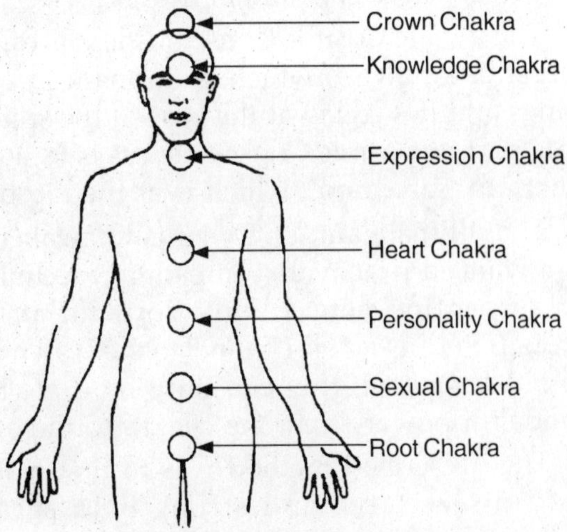

The Seven Body Chakras

Mooladhara Chakra: Root chakra at the base of the spine.

Swadishtana Chakra: Sexual chakra behind the sex organs.

Manipura Chakra: Personality chakra behind the solar plexus.

Anahata Chakra: Heart chakra behind the heart.

Vishudda Chakra: Expressive chakra near the throat.

Ajna Chakra: Knowledge chakra between the eyebrows.

Sahasrara Chakra: Crown chakra near the pituitary gland.

As stated earlier, the chakras are an ancient Hindu concept forming an integral part of Yoga. Patanjali Maharshi propagated Hatha Yoga, also called Ghatasya Yoga (a system of spiritual awakening using the physical body), and Patanjali's *Yoga Sutras* were probably the first text to introduce the concept of chakras.

A chakra is believed to be an energy centre. There are seven chakras placed over the spinal column. These are subtle and cannot be seen through dissection. Yoga believes that the male and female parts of Cosmic Consciousness are present in every human being.

The female Cosmic Consciousness is called *Kundalini* or 'serpentine power', which is dormant in ordinary human beings and lies coiled at the base of the spinal column. The male part of Cosmic Consciousness is located at the crown chakra in 'sahasrara', which is at the top of the head.

The ultimate aim of a yogi is to awaken the Kundalini by advanced pranayama (breathing) techniques and carry the serpentine power lying dormant at the *Mooladhara* through the *Sushumna* channel to the crown chakra. Starting from *Mooladhara*, this can only be done by moving the Kundalini power from one chakra to the other.

The prescribed method was to first make the physical body disease-free and strong by a set of yogasanas. Thereafter, pranayama is practised to awaken the

Kundalini. The awakened Kundalini is then made to rise from one chakra to the other, starting from *Mooladhara* through the *Sushumna nadi*.

The ultimate objective of the yogi is to make the Kundalini reach *Sahasrara*. The union of both then results in the liberation of the soul.

New age spiritualists have more or less accepted the Indian concept of chakras, which has also been recognised by various healing systems developed in Japan and the West.

More importantly, Reiki – a popular form of treatment practised all over the world – deals with therapy through Universal Life Force by supplying the same to chakras, which in turn are supposed to distribute it in the body.

Several other spiritual schools all over the world have also accepted the concept of chakras and believe that their purification can be achieved in various ways and once purified, meditation practices will help in spiritual progress.

Aura healing – another popular holistic healing method practised worldwide – also recognises the role of chakras in health and disease.

Chakra is described as a cone, the apex of which is in contact with the spinal column. The mouth (base) of the cone is about 4 inches in diameter at the end. In other words, the mouth is nearer to the front of the body.

Apart from these seven chakras, several minor chakras are also believed to exist. We will now understand the functioning of each chakra.

1. Root Chakra

The root chakra is the source of our strength and is essential for proper development. It is like the mother of all chakras and controls the functioning of other chakras. In order to do this, the root chakra has to be healthy in the first place. Severe mental and physical problems are caused by disorders in the root chakra.

2. Sexual Chakra

This deals with reproduction. When it is defective, it can lead to kidney, bladder or other problems in connected organs.

3. Personality Chakra

It is located behind the solar plexus and is responsible for proper functioning of the digestive system, liver and gall-bladder.

4. Heart Chakra

It controls the lungs, heart and circulatory system. If this chakra is not functioning properly, these organs are likely to be affected.

5. Expression Chakra

This chakra controls the ability to speak, which is one of the very important and critical functions of existence.

6. Knowledge Chakra

Also called the third-eye chakra or *ajna chakra*, it guides us in a subtle way throughout life. It also determines our approach to life and our spiritual upliftment.

7. Crown Chakra

It is also known as *Sahasrara*. Can be felt and its effect understood only when it is open, which is one of the highest stages of development in Yoga.

While the physical body is connected to all the chakras and the defective chakras can induce disease as mentioned above, on the mental level also chakras have a remarkable influence and determine the behaviour, acceptance levels and the way a person operates in society.

For example, when the root chakra is defective a person may suffer from physical ailments like improper evacuation, piles, fistula, constipation etc. The defective chakra also affects one at the mental level.

When the root chakra is defective, a person becomes aggressive and confused. His aggressive behaviour makes others keep away from him but the person himself is not aware that he is aggressive. The problem with such people is that even when somebody takes pains to explain what is wrong with their behaviour, they hardly understand this, as they are convinced their behaviour is normal.

When defective, the mental aspect of the sexual chakra results in mental withdrawal and creates phobias. Almost all phobias like fear of the dark, fear of being alone, fear of flying, fear of heights, fear of crowds, fear of water, fear of fire, etc, are due to malfunctioning of the chakra at the mental level.

The personality chakra – also called the solar plexus chakra – controls feelings of guilt and shame. When this chakra is defective, the person becomes over-anxious about himself and how society is reacting to him. He is cursed with greed and becomes envious. While taking any action he is always worried about how he is perceived by others and goes out of the way to impress others. Instead of living for himself, he tries to live for others.

The heart chakra interferes with the way a person reacts to people around him. Compassion, kindness, forgiveness and an attitude of give and take are all at the base of this chakra. When this is defective, it makes a person hateful and vengeful.

When the expression chakra or throat chakra is defective, it makes a person unreasonable. This type of person wants everyone to obey him unquestioningly. He becomes a hard taskmaster, but in the process loses the love and respect of others.

The knowledge chakra or ajna chakra is perhaps the most critical one. If this chakra is functioning properly, it will act as a divine guide in the sojourn of life. When this chakra is fully functional, man is completely aware of his activities and responsibilities in life. This chakra guides him in proper planning of life so that progress is continuous and hurdle-free.

When this chakra is defective, a person leads a haphazard life with shifting, inconsistent attitudes and views that ultimately lead him nowhere.

Methods of Administering Colour Therapy

Having understood the role of chakras in disease, we will now look at the various ways in which colour therapy can be administered.

The systems popular all over the world are:

Spot Therapy

Here the desired colour is applied directly over the affected area.

Chakra Therapy

One form of modern colour therapy that is very popular is based on the treatment of chakras to get rid of various ailments. Here the actual area of the body that is affected is not considered important. It is believed that the seat of any disease is the chakra and once the chakra that is associated with the organ is identified, the healing colour is directly administered to this chakra.

Acupuncture Colour Therapy

Another form of colour therapy that is in vogue is the acupuncture form. Acupuncture believes that the origin of the disease is in the meridian, which controls the flow of life energy or *Chi* to the organ. Therefore, the meridian is treated here with colour.

In this case, however, different colours are not used but a single monochromatic light beam is used.

Solarised Water

Colour therapy can also be given in the form of charged water. For this, drinking water is exposed to coloured vibrations and the patient then consumes it. This can be safely given to infants and children as well.

In most cases, colour therapists recommend consumption of solarised water along with chakra healing or the direct exposure method.

Pyramid Colour Healing

Combining pyramid energy with colour is the latest technique of energising colour before the patient receives it.

Pyramid Micro Crystal Cards

Using a technology developed by America's National Aeronautics Space Agency (NASA), Micro Crystal Corporation has developed Pyramid Crystal Cards in different colours, which are applied on the acupuncture points.

We will learn more about all these systems in subsequent chapters.

Spot Application of Colour Therapy

As explained in the preceding chapters, in this method colour vibrations are directly administered to the affected organ of the body.

The Table in this chapter highlights this mode of treatment. The medical term of the disease and a brief explanation for the same is given to facilitate easy understanding.

We will now identify specific diseases connected with various organ systems. The selection of colour sources is dealt with in the next chapter. One could select the source that is convenient and apply the relevant colour.

Head/Eyes/Ears/Nose/Mouth & Throat

Disease	Description	Colour Required	Method of Treatment
Depression	Mental state characterised by excessive sadness.	Yellow	Treat with yellow over the forehead and temples for 15 minutes.
Nervous exhaustion	Fatigued nervous system.	Blue	Treat with blue over the forehead and temples for 15 minutes.
Glaucoma	Progressive loss of vision due to increased pressure in the eyes.	Violet	Violet colour administered to the eyes for an hour daily results in improvement. The best way is to wear a violet-coloured eye-patch while lying down.
Listlessness	Lack of energy, disinterest in life.	Red	Expose yourself to red colour for 10 to 15 minutes.
Mastoiditis	Infection of mastoid bone present near the middle ear resulting in acute pain.	Blue	Treat with blue colour over the ears and behind the neck, just below the ear, for 30 minutes.

Contd...

Disease	Description	Colour Required	Method of Treatment
Mental exhaustion	Feeling mentally tired.	Orange	Treat with orange colour for half an hour daily till relief is obtained.
Migraine	Recurring throbbing headache on one side of the head.	Yellow	To be given above the brow. A glass of yellow solarised water daily is indicated until the condition is under control.
Nightmare	Frightful and terrifying dreams.	Blue	Treat with blue colour over the forehead and temples for 15 minutes.
Night-blindness	Inability to see in insufficient light.	Blue and red	Use blue colour for 15 minutes. For myopia (short-sightedness), use blue light. For distant vision (long-sightedness), use red.
Facial paralysis	A part of the face is drawn to one side.	Yellow and blue	Treat the affected area with yellow colour for 10 minutes, then with blue colour for 10 minutes.

Disease	Description	Colour Required	Method of Treatment
Insanity	Mental disorder.	Blue	Treat with blue on the forehead and temples for 15 minutes.
Insomnia	Inability to have restful sleep.	Blue	Treat with blue colour over the forehead and temples for five minutes. Use more of blue colour in the bedroom.
Chorea or St. Vitus' dance	Disease of the nervous system – induces convulsive movements.	Blue	Treat with blue on front and back of head for 30 minutes daily for about 60 days.
Colds	Infection of respiratory tract.	Red	Treat forehead and temples with red colour for 15 minutes.
Emotional disorders and illness	Catatonic cases where motor abnormalities are associated with mental state.	Blue	Treat with blue colour over the forehead and temples for 15 minutes.

Disease	Description	Colour Required	Method of Treatment
Alzheimer's disease	Mental deterioration similar to senility, occurring in middle age.	Blue, violet and then yellow	Treat the back of the head and crown portions for 10 minutes each.
Baldness	Gradual depletion of hair on the head.	Violet	Treat the scalp in full for 15 minutes daily. More time to be spent on bald patches.
Delirium tremors	In alcoholics, caused by abstinence from alcohol.	Red, blue and yellow	Treat the area around the navel with red for 10 minutes and the forehead with blue for 15 minutes once daily in acute cases; switch to yellow as improvement sets in.
Neurosis	A mental disorder of several types.	Orange	Sitting under orange light or wearing orange clothes till relief is obtained. Use the same colour in bedspreads and curtains for quick recovery.
Blindness	Inability to see due to defect in the eyes.	Green and violet	Where there is no organic damage, use green for 30 minutes twice daily and violet for 20 minutes twice daily, over the neck just below the head.

Disease	Description	Colour Required	Method of Treatment
Dandruff	Disorder of the scalp.	Indigo	Treat with indigo on the scalp for 10 minutes daily before bedtime.
Deafness	Inability to hear properly.	Indigo	Treat with indigo light on top of the head for five minutes; use indigo on back of the head for 10 minutes. Apply indigo on back of the neck for five minutes. Solarised indigo w ater should be taken twice weekly.
Delusion	Baseless fears or beliefs. Examples: the victim thinks he is being followed, stared at, or attempts are being made to poison him.	Blue	Treat with blue light over the forehead and temples for 15 minutes.
Ear ailments	Pain from ear infection or due to exposure to cold wind, ear discharge etc.	Red	Lie on the side and give red colour treatment directly over the affected ear.

Disease	Description	Colour Required	Method of Treatment
Eye inflammation	Red, itching, watery eyes.	Blue	Use blue colour for 15 minutes over closed eyes.
Gum boil	Painful swelling on the gum.	Blue	Treat with blue over the affected tooth. Gargle with solarised water.
Hallucination	Imaginary sightings. Person sees things not seen by others.	Blue	Treat with blue light over the forehead and temples for 15 minutes.
Hysteria	Emotional instability.	Indigo	Treat with indigo on forehead for 15 minutes.
Nose ailments – conditions other than bleeding	Includes allergic conditions.	Violet	Treat with violet colour. Nose bleeding – treat with blue.
Obsession	A form of mental illness where the victim is always nursing thoughts about a single subject.	Green	Exposure to green brings relief. Keep green indoor plants and use green colour in the bedroom.

Disease	Description	Colour Required	Method of Treatment
Parkinson's disease	A slowly progressive disorder of the central nervous system. Characterised by tremor in resting muscles, and by slowness and stiffness of movement. Cause unknown; brain is the seat of disease.	Blue, violet and yellow	Treat affected parts with blue for 30 minutes; follow with violet on top of head and back of head for 15 minutes. In old cases, treat first with yellow for 15 minutes; then follow as above.
Parotid glands	A pair of salivary glands situated in the mouth in front of each ear. Prone to infection, commonly in children.	Blue	Treat with blue light on parotid glands for 10 minutes.
Palsy	A term denoting all types of paralysis.	Green and blue	Treat affected parts with blue and then give green for 10 minutes over affected area.

Disease	Description	Colour Required	Method of Treatment
Earache	Pain in the ear.	Turquoise or light green	Apply for 10 minutes on the affected ear.
Headache	Pain in the head.	Blue and green	Treat the exact location of the pain for 10 minutes with each colour. Blue first. Blue solarised water should be taken daily till the problem ends. Take the treatment lying down with eyes closed so that the colour falls on the entire face.
Toothache	Pain in the teeth.	Blue and violet	Treat the affected part till relief is obtained.
Exophthalmos	Bulging eyeballs.	Blue	Treat the thyroid gland for 15 minutes daily. Drink solarised blue water.
Hoarseness	Skewed voice due to overuse.	Green	Treat with green light for two to three hours daily over voice box; solarised green water is prescribed.
Laryngitis	Loss of voice due to infection.	Indigo	Treat with indigo light on the throat for five minutes; repeat every four hours; drink half glass of blue solarised water every two hours and gargle with the other half.

Disease	Description	Colour Required	Method of Treatment
Meniere's disease	Affects the inner ear. Deafness accompanied by buzzing and giddiness. Cause not known.	Green and violet	Treat with green over the affected ear for 15 minutes each. Treat with violet over the spine for 20 minutes thereafter.
Neuralgia	Severe burning or stabbing pain in the nerve.	Blue	Treat with blue for 10 minutes over kidney area; alternate with orange. If chronic, use yellow in place of orange.
Quinsy sore throat	Pus-filled swelling in the soft palate around the tonsils.	Blue or indigo	Treat with blue or indigo for 20 minutes.
Mental disorders	Emotional disturbance due to shock affecting normal life.	Violet	Treat with violet.
Cataract	Lens of the eye turns opaque.	Indigo	Treat with indigo rays over the affected eye for 10 minutes before bedtime.

Disease	Description	Colour Required	Method of Treatment
Croup	Infection of the larynx in small children.	Violet	Treat with violet colour for 10 minutes.
Granular lid	Inflammation of membrane in the inner lid.	Indigo	Use indigo or blue light for 15 minutes.
Irritation	Losing peace of mind. Annoyance with others.	Indigo	Treat with blue light on the forehead and with indigo on the temple for 15 minutes.
Alponia	Loss of voice due to problem in larynx.	Blue and indigo	Treat with indigo light on the throat for five minutes; repeat every four hours; drink half a glass of blue solarised water every two hours and gargle with the other half.
Scalp	Infection and other skin problems other than dandruff.	Violet	Treat with violet over scalp area for 15 minutes. Applying solarised violet water brings quicker relief.
Tonsillitis	Inflammation of the tonsils.	Violet and blue	Treat with blue light on the throat and with violet on back of neck for 30 minutes.

Disease	Description	Colour Required	Method of Treatment
Torticollis – wryneck	Abnormal twisting of neck resulting in head being held to one side due to excessive muscle contraction.	Blue and green	Treat with blue and green for 10 minutes each over the neck region.
Trifacial neuralgia	Nerves connected with facial expression.	Violet	Treat for 15 minutes on the affected side.
Cerebro-spinal meningitis	Infectious form of meningitis. Inflammation of the membranes of brain and spinal cord due to infection by virus or bacteria causing pneumonia.	Green and violet	Treat with violet over the spine for 20 minutes. Then use green for 15 minutes.
Concussion	Limited period of unconsciousness caused by head injury.	Green and violet	Treat with violet over the head for 20 minutes. Then use green for 10 minutes.

Disease	Description	Colour Required	Method of Treatment
Diphtheria	An infection of the throat.	Green	Treat with green light over the solar plexus, throat and back of neck for 30 minutes every four hours.
Mania	Mental disorder.	Green	Allow the patient to be in a green environment as much as possible. Light green coloured walls in the bedroom and a green bedroom light help.
Epilepsy	A symptom of disorder in the brain; a condition in which seizures occur, leading to convulsions and loss of consciousness.	Blue	Treat with blue light over the head, spine and solar plexus for 20 minutes. Treat abdomen for five minutes. For convulsions, use blue over the occipital area and the spinal cord. Ten minutes on occipital and 20 minutes on spinal cord.
Hay fever	An allergic reaction affecting the nasal cavity. Continuous sneezing, watery discharge.	Yellow and blue	Treat with yellow light on the abdomen for 10 minutes and blue light over the face and chest for 20 minutes.

Disease	Description	Colour Required	Method of Treatment
Hemiplegia	Paralysis of one side of the body. Face and hands are affected more than the legs.	Yellow and indigo	Treat lumbar area with yellow. For paralysis, treat with yellow on back of the neck for 10 minutes, indigo on the spine for 10 minutes, indigo on sacrum and coccyx for 10 minutes. Treat each sciatic nerve with yellow and indigo for 20 minutes.
Hydrophobia	Aversion to water. A sign of rabies.	Blue	Treat with blue light for two to three hours daily; solarised water is also prescribed.
Iritis	Infection of the iris.	Blue	Treat with blue over the eyes for 30 minutes.
Measles	Infectious disease normally affecting children.	Yellow, blue and red	First treat with yellow and red, then follow with blue over torso for 20 minutes.
Mumps	Infectious disease, usually occurring in childhood, marked by swelling of the large salivary glands in front of the ears.	Blue	Treat with blue light just below the ears for 10 minutes.

Disease	Description	Colour Required	Method of Treatment
Myocarditis	Acute inflammation of the heart muscle.	Red and blue	Treat with red rays to stimulate the heart. Treat with blue rays to calm the heart.
Nose bleeding	Normally due to rupture of small blood vessels.	Indigo	Treat with indigo until it stops.
Mouth ulcers	Eruptions inside the mouth on skin surface.	Violet	Treat mouth with violet for 15 minutes. Solarised water mouthwash prescribed.
Multiple sclerosis	Chronic, progressive, degenerative disease of central nervous system.	Indigo	Treat the entire body for 30 minutes.
Sinusitis	Inflammation of nasal sinuses.	Green and blue	Treat with green for 10 minutes behind the neck and head and blue on sinus for 10 minutes.
Smell deficiency	Inability to smell or differentiate odours.	Indigo	Treat face and head with indigo for 15 minutes.

Disease	Description	Colour Required	Method of Treatment
Sore throat	Throat infection caused by specific bacteria.	Indigo and blue	Treat with indigo or blue for 20 minutes.
Tetanus or lockjaw	A serious infection caused by bacteria that enter open wounds.	Violet	Treat nervous system with violet for 30 minutes four times daily.
Vertigo	Giddiness, losing balance while walking.	Indigo	Treat with indigo light on top of the head for five minutes; use indigo behind the head for 10 minutes and indigo on back of neck for five minutes. Solarised water prescribed twice weekly. If emotional in origin, also treat emotions.

Chest/Heart/Back

Disease	Description	Colour Required	Method of Treatment
Back pain	A regular complaint in middle age due to bad posture. Not related to prolapsed discs.	Blue and green	Treat the entire length of the spinal column with blue colour, concentrating more on the painful spot. Treat the lower back with green colour after the application of blue.
Mastitis	Inflammation of the breasts. Normally caused by fissures in nipples. Sometimes internal infection occurs without involvement of nipples.	Blue	Treat with blue light over the affected breast for 10 minutes. Continue treatment with blue light on ovaries for 10 minutes. Drink blue solarised water daily till improvement occurs.
Pain in the lower back	Due to muscular strain.	Green	Use green on small of back and lower back.
Angina pectoris	Pain in the centre of the chest.	Red and blue	Treat with red rays to stimulate the heart. Treat with blue rays to calm the heart.

Disease	Description	Colour Required	Method of Treatment
Angina and pseudo-angina	A choking, suffocating sense of pain in the chest area, mimicking angina pains but not related to heart ailment. Mainly of psychosomatic origin.	Red and blue	Red rays to stimulate the heart. Blue rays to calm the heart. For 10 minutes each.
Aortitis	Inflammation of the aorta.	Blue or green	Treat for 20 minutes with blue or green on the chest area near the painful spot.
Asthma	Difficulty in breathing due to narrowing of air passages.	Red, yellow, indigo, violet and orange	In adults, red, yellow, or orange can be used. If the system is emaciated, use red one day and yellow the following day. After an attack, use orange. Solarised water is always indicated. In acute stage, indigo or violet is mandatory. Treat for 15 minutes on chest and upper back.
Cardiac asthma	Related to insufficient flow of blood to the lungs.	Red	Treat with red for 10 minutes on abdomen.
Asthma in children	Normally due to allergens in the air.	Red	Use red on pancreas – a gland that lies behind the stomach and produces insulin.

Disease	Description	Colour Required	Method of Treatment
Heartburn	A disease due to bad digestion. Gases cause burning sensation in the chest region below the heart.	Purple	Treat with purple light over the abdomen for 15 minutes. Solarised water should be taken daily.
Hiccups	Sharp, repeated sound caused by contractions of the diaphragm.	Blue	Treat with blue light on the throat for five minutes; repeat every four hours. Drink half a glass of blue solarised water every two hours and gargle with the other half.
Breast pain	Normally felt during menstruation cycles.	Pink, red and violet	Apply each colour for five minutes. First pink, followed by red and then violet.
Lumbago	Low back pain.	Yellow and blue	Treat with yellow light on abdomen for 15 minutes; treat with blue light on lower back and the end of the spinal column for 15 minutes.

Disease	Description	Colour Required	Method of Treatment
Breast tumour	Growth or painless hard swelling in the breast region.	Indigo, green, orange and violet	Alternate use of indigo and green or orange, using each colour on alternate days, minimum 20 minutes. Also treat the spine for 10 minutes. Treat the pituitary, thyroid, adrenal cortex, and ovaries for five minutes each in that order. Treat abdomen just over the navel and three inches on either side of midline for five minutes. Treat pancreas for five minutes. Finish with violet light on forehead and temples for five minutes each.
Amyotrophic lateral sclerosis	Disease causing paralysis due to degeneration of spinal cord.	Blue and yellow	Treat the nervous system with blue for 15 minutes in acute cases. Treat the extremities with yellow for 10 minutes and then follow with blue to treat the nervous system. For chronic cases, twice daily.
Endocarditis and myocarditis	Endocarditis – inflammation of inner lining of the heart, especially the heart valves. Myocarditis – inflammation of the heart muscle.	Blue and red	Treat with red rays to stimulate the heart and with blue rays to calm the heart.

Disease	Description	Colour Required	Method of Treatment
Lung congestion	Lungs filled with mucus.	Violet	Treat with violet for 10 minutes.
Phleginatic fever	Fever due to congestion in lungs. Person coughs and brings out phlegm.	Blue	Treat with blue light front and back, 15 minutes each.
Pneumonia	Infection of the lungs.	Indigo, red and orange	Treat with indigo on upper chest for 30 minutes. Make sure the light hits the sternum on second rib. In acute cases, treat with indigo, solarised water, and light. In chronic cases, use charged red or orange water. Treat upper chest on sternum for 10 minutes.
Whooping cough	Caused by infection. Mostly affects children.	Violet and blue	Treat with blue or violet light on chest and upper back for 30 minutes twice daily, for a week to ten days.
Low blood pressure	Blood pressure falls below normal.	Red and orange	Use red and orange over the heart area for 10 minutes each.

Disease	Description	Colour Required	Method of Treatment
Bronchitis or pneumonia	Bronchitis – inflammation of the bronchi due to various bacteria and narrowing of bronchi causing difficulty in breathing.	Indigo, red and orange	In acute cases, treat with indigo, solarised water, and light; in chronic cases, use red or orange water and light. Treat upper chest or front chest bone for 10 minutes.
Coughs	Irritation in the airways causing violent exhalation.	Indigo and orange	For dry cough, treat with indigo, solarised water and light on chest for 10 minutes. For wet cough, substitute orange light and orange solarised water.
Dropsy	Collection of fluid in the body.	Blue	Treat with blue light on the affected part.
Stenosis, cardiac dilation and bradycardia	Narrowing of the passage carrying blood.	Red	Use scarlet red for 10 to 15 minutes.
Circulation disease	Blood circulation disorders, insufficient supply of blood to any organ resulting in swelling.	Red	Treat with red rays to stimulate the heart.

Disease	Description	Colour Required	Method of Treatment
High blood pressure	Higher pressure exerted on arterial valves resulting in strain on the heart.	Blue or green	Use light blue or green.
Palpitation	Rapid pulsation of the heart.	Blue, red and yellow	Use blue over the heart, red over the solar plexus and yellow over the abdomen.
Hypertension	High blood pressure in the arteries.	Blue	Treat with blue light over the forehead and temples for 15 minutes.
Hyperthyroidism	Excessive activity of the thyroid.	Blue	Treat with blue colour on the thyroid for 15 minutes daily. Have a glass of solarised water daily.
Tuberculosis	An infectious disease of the lungs that can be fatal.	Yellow, orange, violet, turquoise and blue	Treat with orange over the chest and back for 30 minutes, then violet for 10 minutes. If constipated, use yellow over abdomen; finish with light colour over forehead and temples for three minutes each. Turquoise is specified when fever is present. If fever increases, switch to blue.

Abdominal/Digestive/Kidney/Urinary Organs

Disease	Description	Colour Required	Method of Treatment
Colic	Acute pain in the abdomen and bowels.	Yellow	Treat with yellow on abdomen and drink yellow solarised water, except for inflammation and diarrhoea.
Constipation	Difficulty in evacuation.	Yellow	For constipation, use yellow for 10 minutes. A glass of yellow solarised water daily is indicated until the condition improves. Take proper diet that is easily digestible and has more fibre.
Colitis	Inflammation of the mucous membrane of the colon.	Yellow, blue and green	Use yellow for 10 minutes. For diarrhoea, use blue or green. A glass of yellow solarised water daily is prescribed until the condition is under control. Carefully control the diet during treatment.

Contd...

Disease	Description	Colour Required	Method of Treatment
Dyspepsia	Impaired power of digestion.	Yellow	Treat abdominal region for 15 minutes daily. And drink yellow solarised water.
Stomach ailments	Pain in the abdominal region.	Yellow	Treat for 15 minutes in the painful area. Also drink yellow solarised water.
Duodentis	An ulcer in the duodenum.	Blue	Administer blue for 15 minutes over the area. Also drink blue solarised water.
Haemorrhoids	Enlarged veins in the walls of the anus.	Blue and red	Apply red in the neck portion at the back just below the head for 10 minutes. Simultaneously apply blue at the end of the spinal column. Drink blue solarised water.
Jaundice	A liver disease caused by viral infection.	Blue	Treat with blue light over the fifth rib on the right side in the midline for five to ten minutes.
Indigestion	Indigestion and pain or discomfort in upper abdominal area after eating, accompanied by nausea and vomiting.	Yellow	Treat with yellow on abdomen and drink yellow solarised water till recovery.

Disease	Description	Colour Required	Method of Treatment
Stomach-ache	Pain in the lower and upper intestinal area.	Yellow	Treat with yellow on abdomen and have yellow solarised water, except for inflammations and diarrhoea.
Prostate condition	A small gland found behind the bladder in males. Prone to enlargement in old age, causing difficulty in urination.	Indigo, green and orange	Treat with indigo over the prostate area, then treat bladder. For prostate cancer, alternate use of indigo and green or orange, using each colour on alternate days. Treat spine for 10 minutes. Treat the pituitary, thyroid, adrenal cortex, ovaries or prostate for five minutes each in that order. Treat abdomen just over navel and three inches on either side of midline for five minutes. Treat pancreas for five minutes. Finish with indigo light on forehead and temples, five minutes each.
Urethritis	Urethritis is the inflammation of urethra normally due to gonorrhoea or insertion of catheter in aged people.	Blue, green and yellow	For gonorrhoea, treat with blue light over lower back and genitals for 45 minutes daily for two to six weeks. Every three days use green instead of blue. For re-infection, use yellow. For bladder, treat with blue; alternate with yellow over the lower spine for 10 minutes. Drink a glass of solarised blue water daily. For incontinence, use green or purple light.

Disease	Description	Colour Required	Method of Treatment
Pain in the gall-bladder	A pear-shaped sac behind the first lobe of the liver that stores and delivers bile.	Orange, yellow, blue and green	Treat with orange for 10 minutes in the affected area. For constipation, use yellow for 10 minutes. For diarrhoea, use blue or green. A glass of solarised water a day is indicated until the condition is under control. Check the diet also.
Gall-stones	A hard mass comprising bile pigments, cholesterol and calcium, formed in the gall-bladder.	Orange	Treat with orange light on the abdomen about three inches above the navel for 15 minutes; drink orange solarised water.
Anorexia	Lack of appetite.	Blue	Treat with blue over the umbilical area for 10 minutes.
Excessive appetite	Irresistible urge to eat.	Indigo	Apply over the abdomen for 15 minutes before meal-time.
Belching	Undigested food matter coming to the mouth.	Yellow	Treat the abdominal area for 15 minutes before eating, morning and evening.

Disease	Description	Colour Required	Method of Treatment
Loss of appetite	Lack of desire for food.	Yellow	Apply over the abdomen for 15 minutes before meal-time.
Digestive ailments	Ailments associated with improper digestion and malfunctioning of any of the various associated organs.	Yellow	Treat with yellow on abdomen and yellow solarised water, except for inflammation and diarrhoea.
Bladder inflammation and incontinence	The bladder is a sac-like organ storing urine. Incontinence is the inability to control discharge of urine.	Violet, blue, yellow and green	Treat with blue and alternate with yellow over the lower spine for 10 minutes. Have a glass of solarised blue water. For incontinence, use green or violet light.

Disease	Description	Colour Required	Method of Treatment
Renal insufficiency	Kidneys malfunction and fail to purify the blood properly.	Violet and orange	Treat with violet light for 10 minutes over the kidney area. Alternate with orange.
Kidney stones	Stones in kidney formed from body salts blocking passages and causing acute pain.	Orange	Treat with orange light for 15 minutes and drink orange solarised water regularly, till pain subsides and urine discharge is normal.
Bright's disease	Inflammation of the kidney. Varied causes.	Indigo and orange	Treat with indigo light for 10 minutes over the kidney area. Alternate with orange.
Cystitis – acute, chronic	Inflammation of urinary bladder mostly due to infection. Burning pain often accompanied by blood while passing urine.	Blue, yellow, green and purple	Treat with blue and alternate with yellow over the lower spine for 10 minutes. Have a glass of solarised blue water. For incontinence, use green or purple light.
Amoebic dysentery	Infectious form of diarrhoea.	Indigo and blue	Treat abdominal area and lower back for 15 minutes each. Consume blue solarised water.

Disease	Description	Colour Required	Method of Treatment
Abdominal cramps	Pain in the abdominal region.	Yellow	Treat the area for 15 minutes.
Weak liver	Insufficient bile secretion resulting in improper digestion.	Blue, yellow, orange and green	Treat the liver with blue light over the fifth rib on the right side in the midline for five minutes. If accompanied by constipation, use yellow for 10 minutes. If accompanied by diarrhoea, use blue or green. Have a glass of blue solarised water daily until the condition is under control. Diet should be checked. For gall-bladder, treat the affected area with orange for 10 minutes.
Biliousness	A liver disorder.	Blue	Treat for 15 minutes twice daily over the liver area.
Hepatitis	Inflammation of the liver due to presence of toxic substances or infection caused by viruses.	Blue	Treat with blue light over the liver for 15 minutes, twice daily.

Disease	Description	Colour Required	Method of Treatment
Cholera	A gut infection. Causes violent vomiting and diarrhoea.	Violet	Treat with violet on abdomen for 30 minutes twice daily.
Liver cirrhosis	A condition in which the liver forms fibrous tissues in strands. Due to excessive alcohol consumption.	Blue	Treat with blue light over the fifth rib on the right side in the midline for 45 minutes.
Dehydration	Fall in the water content of tissues much below normal, due to purging or vomiting.	Blue	Treat with blue for 20 minutes over the abdomen. Give solarised water frequently.
Diarrhoea	Loose motions or watery stools.	Blue and yellow	Treat with blue light over abdomen for 30 minutes. Give one glass of yellow solarised water daily.

Disease	Description	Colour Required	Method of Treatment
Hyper-acidity	Excessive acid formation in stomach.	Green	Treat abdominal area for 10 minutes, twice daily.
Hypo-acidity	Shortage of acid in the stomach.	Green	Treat abdominal area for 10 minutes, twice daily.
Diverticulitis	Inflammation of small pouches in large intestine. Pain in the lower abdomen with constipation or diarrhoea.	Yellow, blue or green	For constipation, use yellow for 10 minutes. For diarrhoea, use blue or green. A glass of solarised water a day is prescribed until the condition is under control.
Duodenal ulcer	Inflammation of the duodenum.	Blue	Treat with blue light on abdominal area for 30 minutes; blue light on forehead and temples for three minutes each. Solarised water, one glass daily.

Disease	Description	Colour Required	Method of Treatment
Gastric ulcer	Erosion of the stomach mucous caused by acid and bile.	Yellow and green	Treat with yellow light over the abdomen and lower back for 15 minutes each. Apply green light on forehead and temples for three minutes.
Gastrointestinal ailments	Diseases in stomach intestine.	Yellow	Treat with yellow light on abdomen and yellow solarised water, except for inflammations and diarrhoea.
Hyperchlorhydria	Greater than normal secretion of hydrochloric acid in the stomach often leading to ulcers.	Blue	Treat with blue light for 20 minutes on stomach.
Hypermotility of the G.I. tract	Excessive movement of the stomach and intestinal tract.	Blue	Treat with blue light for 20 minutes on stomach.
Peritonitis	Inflammation of the sac holding the abdominal organs.	Blue and indigo	Treat with blue and indigo for 20 minutes.

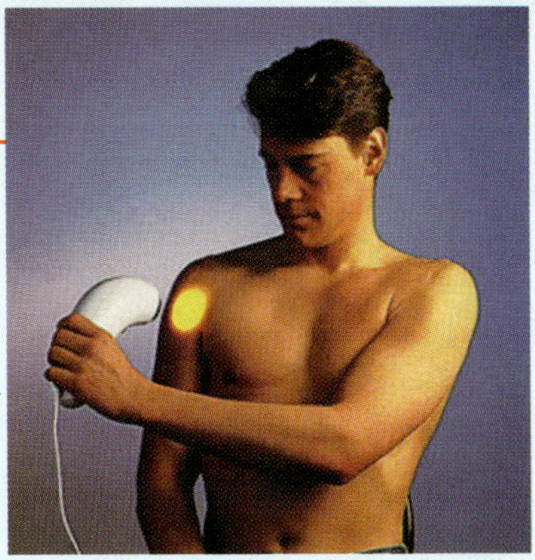

A patient using yellowlight treatment (*see page 73*).

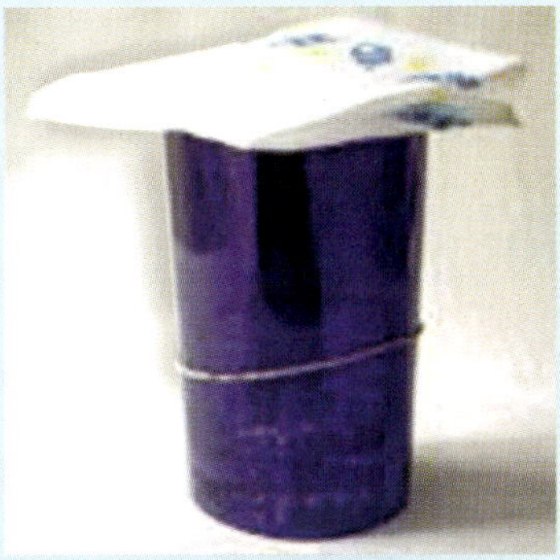

A glass of solarised water (*see page 31*).

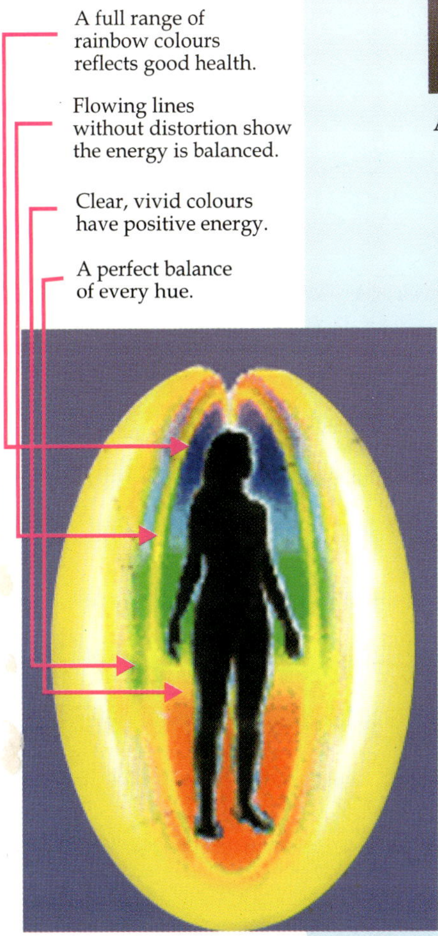

Colours can affect a person's aura (*see page 27*).

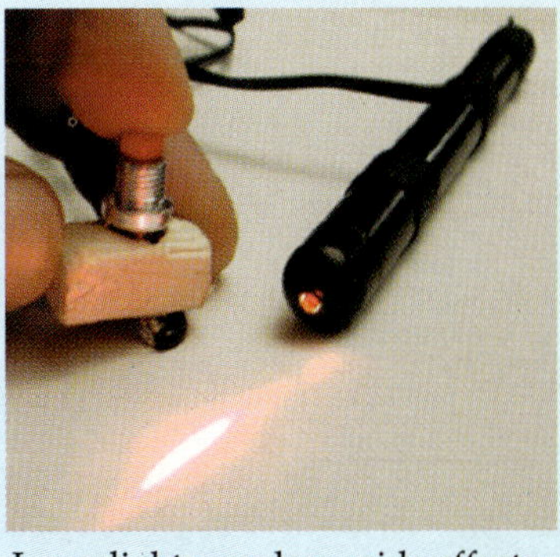

Laser lights can have side effects (*see page 105*).

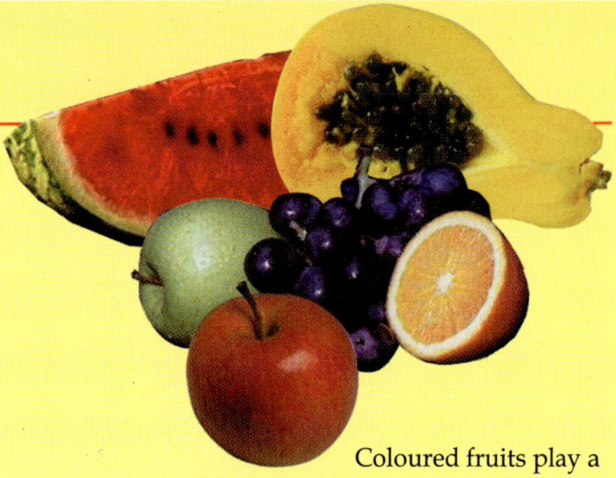

Coloured fruits play a role in colour therapy (*see pages 88 & 89*).

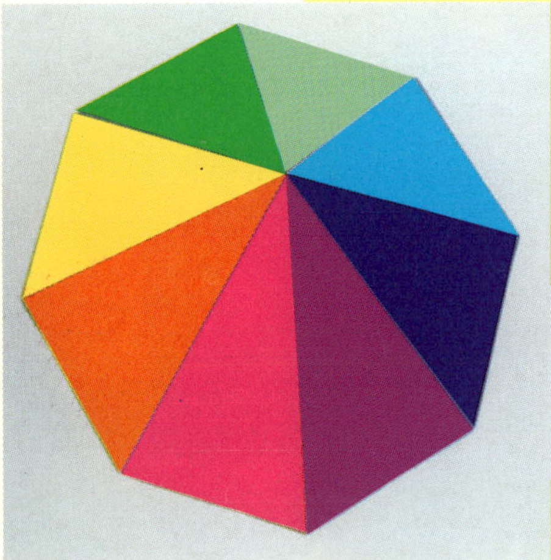

An octagonal pyramid with eight colours (*see page 110*).

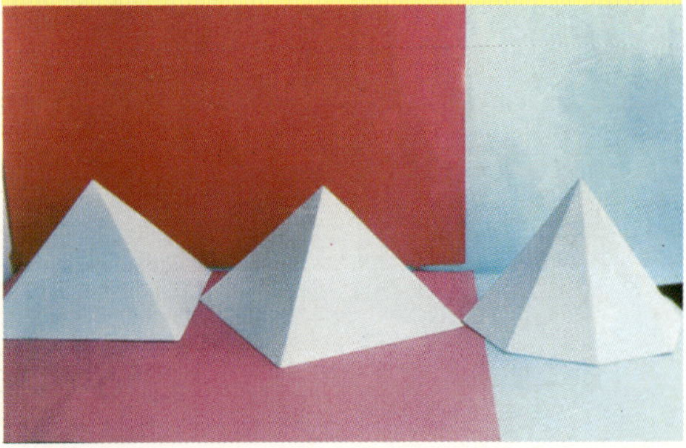

Four-cornered and octagonal pyramids (*see page 110*).

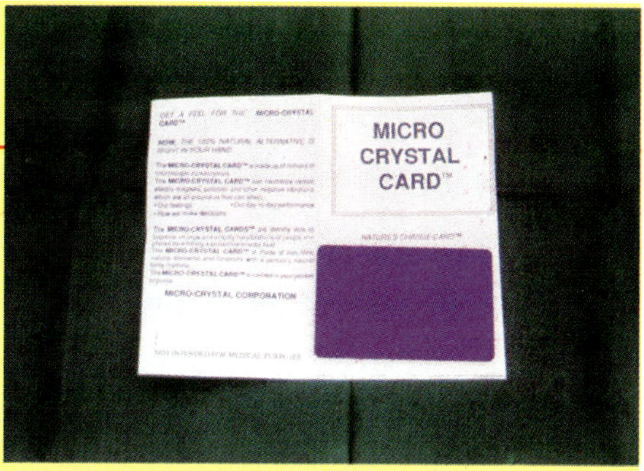

A micro-crystal card (*see pages 118 & 119*).

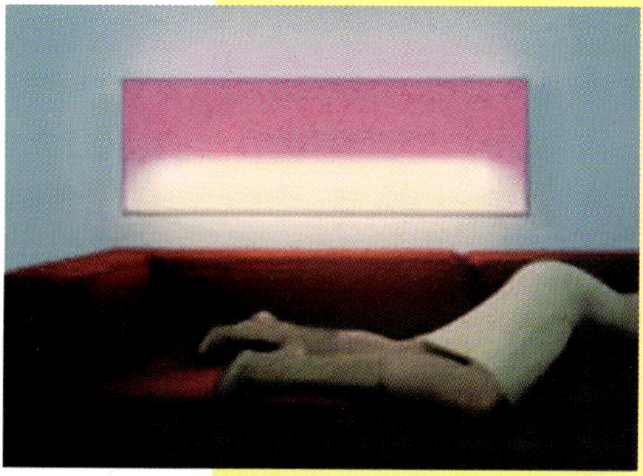

A room with lighting for colour therapy (*see page 15*).

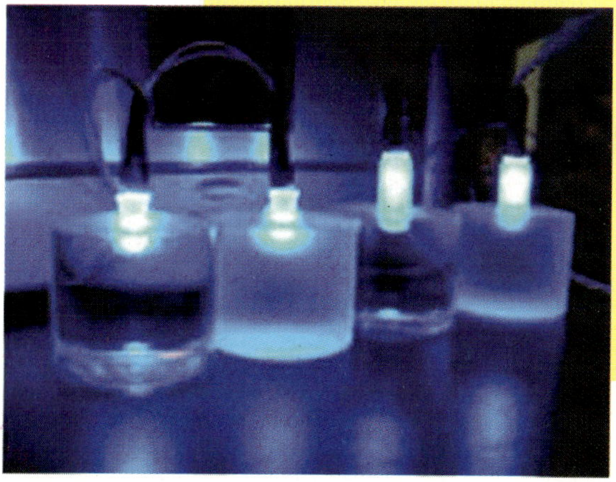

LED lights are one source of coloured lights (*see page 105*).

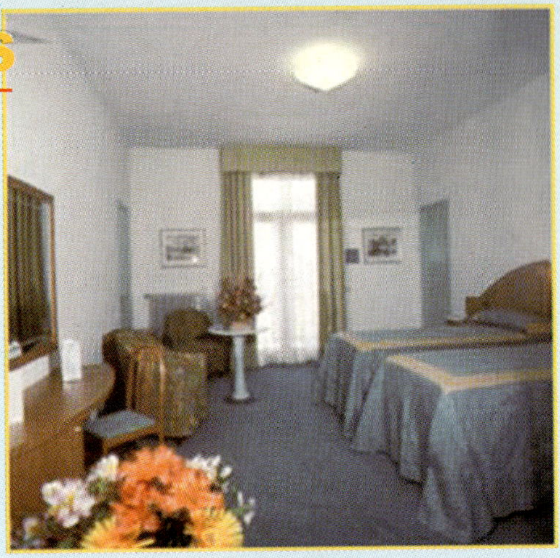

Sky blue colour in the bedroom is beneficial in typhoid (*see page 65*).

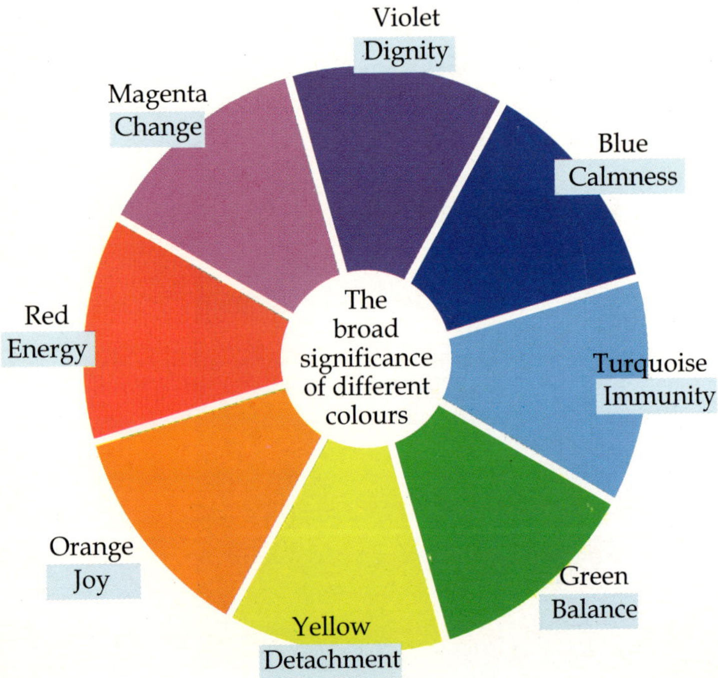

(*see pages 13, 87 & 88*)

Disease	Description	Colour Required	Method of Treatment
Typhoid	Fever caused by infection. Water-borne disease.	Blue	Use plenty of sky blue colour in the patient's bedroom.
Vomiting	Reflex action whereby stomach contents are thrown up violently.	Blue	Treat with blue over navel area every three hours for 10 minutes.

Reproductive Organs

Disease	Description	Colour Required	Method of Treatment
Amenorrhoea	Absence of menstruation in girls of marriageable age.	Blue	Treat with blue for 10 minutes each on sacrum, on the lower part of abdomen right and left side, and the thyroid.
Dysmenorrhoea in young women	Painful or difficult menstruation.	Blue	Treatment can be given during menses. Start with blue colour for 10 minutes each on left and right side of lower abdomen. Another 10 minutes of blue colour treatment over the thyroid, as the malfunctioning of the thyroid gland causes this problem.
Frigidity	Lack of sexual desire in women.	Blue and orange	Treat lower abdominal area involving the reproductive organs with blue for 15 minutes daily. After this, treat only ovaries with orange for 10 minutes on each side.
Inflammation of gonads	The reproductive organs in male/female are called gonads.	Violet and blue	Treat the genital organ with violet colour twice daily for minimum 30 minutes each till relief is obtained. Drink blue solarised water daily.
Cessation of menstruation	Stopping of menstrual flow.	Orange	Treat with orange for 20 minutes.
Orchitis	Inflammation of testicles.	Blue	Treat with blue over the groin and testicles for 30 minutes.
Ovarian pain	Pain in the region of the ovary.	Blue	Treat with blue light for 10 minutes.

Disease	Description	Colour Required	Method of Treatment
Ovarian cysts	A sac filled with fluid that forms in the ovary.	Orange, indigo and green	Use indigo and green or orange on alternate days. Treat the spine for 10 minutes just over the navel and three inches on either side of the midline for five minutes.
Sterility	Inability to bear children.	Indigo	Treat base of sacrum (a curved triangular element of the backbone above the coccyx) with indigo for half-hour.
Vomiting during pregnancy	–	Indigo or violet	Treat with indigo or violet for 15 minutes daily.
Impotence	Inability to have or sustain an erection.	Yellow and indigo	Treat with yellow on small of back for 15 minutes, then with indigo for 15 minutes.
Menopause	End of a woman's reproductive life, marked by symptoms like hot flashes and irritability.	Green and yellow	Treat with green for 20 minutes over ovaries, yellow for 10 minutes over kidney, and green for 10 minutes over the forehead.
Syphilis	Sexually transmitted disease.	Green, blue and yellow	Treat with green and blue light over spinal cord and chest for 20 minutes daily for several weeks. Then switch to yellow for several weeks. Solarised water is prescribed.

Extremities

Disease	Description	Colour Required	Method of Treatment
Milk leg	Swelling of the leg due to a clot. Normally experienced by women after childbirth.	Blue and yellow	Treat with blue light at the back of the neck and affected part for 20 minutes. Alternate every day with yellow.
Synovitis	Inflammation of the lining of a joint leading to acute pain. May arise due to infection or arthritis.	Yellow and blue	Treat affected part for ten minutes alternately with yellow and blue.
Intermittent claudication	Pain experienced in calf and leg muscles after exercise or walking.	Red, blue and green	Treat affected area with blue for 20 minutes. Treat with red if no fever is present; use orange if patient suffers from hypertension. Green on head and blue on chest if fever or inflammation is present.

Disease	Description	Colour Required	Method of Treatment
Elbow tenderness	Pain in the elbows.	Violet and blue	Treat affected area with violet. Treat pancreas with blue.
Paralysis	Progressive weakness in different parts of the body. Severity depends on the areas affected.	Yellow and indigo	Treat with yellow on back of neck for 10 minutes, indigo on spine for 10 minutes, indigo on testicles and end of spinal column for 10 minutes. Treat each sciatic nerve with yellow and indigo for 20 minutes.
Infantile paralysis	Paralysis in infants.	Indigo and red	Treat with indigo for 30 minutes over the spine. Repeat thrice daily. Treat pancreas with red.
Brachial neuritis	Inflammation of nerves in the upper arm.	Violet	To be applied over the affected area for 30 minutes twice daily.

Disease	Description	Colour Required	Method of Treatment
Gout	Disease in which there is an upset in the metabolism of uric acid, causing symptoms of joint pain.	Violet, orange and blue	Treat with orange over abdomen for 10 minutes and blue over the toes and wrists for 15 minutes. Finish with violet.
Knee trouble	Pain while sitting or standing.	Orange, blue and green	Treat affected area with orange for 10' minutes. If due to gonorrhoea – treat with blue light over lumbars and genital organs, 45 minutes daily for two to six weeks. Every three days use green instead of blue.
Rheumatism	A form of arthritis involving joints of fingers, fists, legs and ankles. Sometimes hip and shoulder joints too.	Orange, blue and green	If acute, use blue or green solarised water and light on affected parts for 30 minutes. If chronic, substitute orange.

Disease	Description	Colour Required	Method of Treatment
Raynaud's disease	A disease where the arteries of extremities are unduly active and create spasm. Cause unknown.	Red and blue	Treat with red light for 20 minutes on hands and toes in the morning. Give blue in the evening. Duration: 30 minutes.
Apoplexy (stroke)	A sudden attack of paralysis affecting one side of the body.	Blue	Treat with blue on forehead right over the frontal protuberances.
Pain in bones	Pain due to nerves touching bones.	Violet and yellow	Treat affected area with violet followed by yellow. Violet soothes pain, while yellow energises.
Sciatica	Pain in the sciatic nerve, felt in the back of the thigh, leg and foot.	Yellow and blue	Treat with yellow light on abdomen for 15 minutes and with blue light on lower lumbar and sacrum for 15 minutes.

Muscles

Disease	Description	Colour Required	Method of Treatment
Muscle ache	Commonly caused by strain and tearing of muscle.	Orange	Treat affected area with orange for 30 minutes, twice daily.
Angina and hypertrophy	Hypertrophy is an increase in the size of an organ due to increase in the size of its constituent cells.	Magenta	Magenta reinforces the heart action. It also has the same rate of vibration as lethiumin, potassium, strontium and manganese. Known to energise the heart.
Spasm	Sustained involuntary muscular contraction.	Blue	Use blue solarised water, twice daily.
Cramps	Muscular contraction resulting in pain.	Green and blue	Apply for 15 minutes over the affected area.

Skin Disorders

Disease	Description	Colour Required	Method of Treatment
Dry skin	A condition in which moisture content of the skin is below normal.	Yellow and orange	Apply for 15 minutes over the affected area.
Excessively oily skin	Condition in which the skin's oil glands are overactive.	Green and blue	Treat with each colour for 15 minutes.
Moles	A dark brown area on the skin, which can be flat or raised. Sometimes leads to malignancy.	Red	Treat for 15 minutes over the mole.
Blisters	Watery fluid under the skin. Common in burn injuries. Sometimes formed due to allergic reaction of chemicals, especially sulphur compounds.	Blue	Treat with blue colour for 15 minutes and soak with blue solarised water.

Contd...

Disease	Description	Colour Required	Method of Treatment
Leprosy	A skin disease that leads to the loss of extremities if untreated.	Red and yellow	Treat with yellow and red over the affected parts for 30 minutes twice daily.
Leucoderma (pigmentation disease)	White patches over the skin, caused by the inability of cells to make pigment. Not infectious.	Blue	Treat affected area with blue.
Abscesses	Pus formation – localised infection.	Violet	If internal, treat with solarised water. If external, wash with solarised water and give colour therapy for 15 minutes twice daily.
Acne	A skin disorder in adolescents.	Orange	The same as above.
Itching	A skin condition prompting scratching for relief.	Blue	Treat the affected area with blue for 10 minutes.
Boils and carbuncles	Boils: tender inflamed area of the skin filled with pus. Carbuncles: collection of boils with multiple draining channels.	Yellow and orange	Treat with yellow on abdomen just over the navel and three inches on either side of the midline for one minute. Treat with orange locally for 20 minutes. Drink solarised yellow water.

Disease	Description	Colour Required	Method of Treatment
Bruises	An area of skin discoloration caused by the escape of blood from ruptured underlying vessels following injury.	Violet	Treat with violet for 15 minutes twice daily.
Burns	Scalding of skin due to direct contact with fire.	Blue and green	Alternate blue and green colour over the affected part.
Chicken pox	Itchy rash appears on the skin, which consists of fluid-filled blisters.	Green	Treat with green light on torso for 30 minutes on each side.
Erysipelas	Bacterial infection of the skin and underlying tissues, usually on face and scalp.	Red and blue	Treat with red for 10 minutes and blue for 15 minutes.
Lupus	Tuberculosis of the skin.	Blue	Treat with blue over the affected part for 30 minutes; drink solarised water.
Urticaria	Uncontrollable itching of the skin due to infection.	Green	Treat the affected area with green for 10 minutes.

Blood Disorders

Disease	Description	Colour Required	Method of Treatment
Haemorrhage	Escape of blood from a ruptured blood vessel.	Blue	Treat with blue light over the affected area till bleeding stops.
Anaemia	Reduction in haemoglobin levels.	Red	Treat with red light bath for 10 minutes daily, concentrating on upper back for five minutes. Drink a glass of red solarised water daily.
Blood ailments	Blood diseases.	Red	Treat with red.
Cholorsis (greenish colour of skin)	Severe form of anaemia produced by gross deficiency of iron.	Red	Treat with red light bath for 10 minutes daily, concentrating on the spinal column. Drink a glass of red solarised water daily.

Disease	Description	Colour Required	Method of Treatment
Enlargement of spleen	A large dark organ situated behind and below the stomach, responsible for keeping blood healthy.	Orange	Treat with orange colour over spleen area for half an hour.
Diabetes	A disorder resulting in accumulation of sugar in blood and urine.	Yellow	Treat over pancreas for 15 minutes.
Bleeding	Oozing of blood from an organ or body part.	Indigo and blue	Treat nose ailments with indigo until it stops. Treat haemorrhage with blue over the affected area.
Leukaemia	Blood cancer.	Green, indigo and orange	Use indigo and green or orange on alternate days.

General Ailments

Disease	Description	Colour Required	Method of Treatment
Fistula	An abnormal passage leading from the surface of the body to an internal cavity.	Blue and indigo	Treat with blue light for 10 minutes and with indigo for 10 minutes.
AIDS (Acquired Immune Deficiency Syndrome)	A fatal disease caused by the HIV virus, primarily transmitted through sex.	Red, indigo and violet, followed by pink and gold.	Treat for 15 minutes with each colour.
Undiagnosed fevers	Fevers caused by unknown agents.	Blue	Treat with blue for 15 minutes each on back and front, four times daily.
Alcoholism	An addictive disease marked by a craving for alcohol.	Red and blue	Treat the area around the navel with red for 10 minutes and the forehead with blue for 15 minutes.
Allergies	Abnormal sensitivity to any substance.	Indigo and orange	Alternate treatment with indigo and orange for 10 minutes over the affected area.

Disease	Description	Colour Required	Method of Treatment
Debility	Weakness	Violet	Treat with violet on forehead.
Scurvy	A disease caused by vitamin C deficiency. Appears as black patches over the skin.	Blue	Treatment over the spine with blue.
Malaria	An infectious disease marked by recurrent bouts of fever and chills.	Blue and yellow	Treat with blue during feverish state and yellow during chill. Blue to be used on head area.
Rickets	Disease affecting children due to vitamin D deficiency. Bones do not harden but get deformed.	Blue	Treat with blue colour on chest for 20 minutes.
Rounded shoulders in children	Disorder due to weak ribs resulting in a circular ribcage and rounded shoulders.	Yellow	Solarised water to be consumed daily.
Shock	Acute circulatory failure, when the arterial blood pressure is too low to provide normal blood supply to the body.	Blue, indigo and red	Treat with blue light on back of neck for 10 minutes and indigo on upper chest area for 20 minutes. Treat extremities with red.

Disease	Description	Colour Required	Method of Treatment
Cancer	Any malignant tumour.	Indigo, green and orange	Treat with indigo and green or orange, using each on alternate days.
Character changes	Sudden change in the behaviour of a person.	Blue	Treat with blue light over the forehead and temple for 15 minutes.
Cysts (except ovarian)	A sac containing morbid matter.	Green	Treat with green over the affected area.
Inflammation	The response of the body's tissues to injury, which involves pain, heat, redness and swelling.	Green and blue	Treat with blue generally and green locally.

Disease	Description	Colour Required	Method of Treatment
Tumour	An abnormal swelling in any part of the body consisting of an unusual growth of tissue, possibly malignant.	Green, indigo and orange	Treat with indigo and green or orange, using each colour on alternate days.
Typhus	A serious infection. High fever, headache, rashes and delirium are main symptoms. Believed to be caused by ticks on rats.	Blue and green	Treat with blue light over spinal cord for 30 minutes every four hours, followed by green.
Wounds	A sudden break in body tissue and/or organs caused by an external agent.	Violet	Treat with violet on wound. Depending on the extent and severity of wound, the time will vary from 10 minutes to an hour.
Yellow fever	A type of infectious fever caused by mosquitoes.	Blue and yellow	Treat with blue light on the head and yellow light on the abdomen.

Interchanging Colours

Sometimes, you may find a colour too strong, although as far as its effect on the cure is concerned, you may get beneficial results. In such cases, it is wiser to alternate the colour with another colour, which can be interchanged.

For example, if red is recommended for a particular ailment, and if red is too strong for you, use orange or yellow. Similarly, orange can be interchanged with yellow and red.

At the end of the spectrum, blue, indigo and violet are interchangeable. Similarly, wherever green is recommended, if the effect is not satisfactory, try blue.

Sources of Colour

In the last chapter, we have dwelt on the application of colours to treat various ailments. This chapter outlines the various methods of imparting colour therapy. We need a source for the desired colour if the treatment is to be administered.

Here are the various colour sources utilised in colour therapy.

Coloured Electrical Bulbs

Most colours can be imparted by various means. Coloured glass bulbs are one of the easiest and most effective means of adding colour.

Normally, these bulbs are available in various colours like red, blue, green, orange, yellow, etc. Do not buy a bulb with light coloured glass where you can see the filament. You should buy clouded bulbs like the ones made by Philips, where only coloured light is emitted and one cannot see the filament.

Fluorescent lamps and neon lamps are not recommended, as these are unhealthy. If anybody in the house is suffering from frequent health problems due to seasonal changes, do not use fluorescent lamps in their bedrooms.

Any colour that is used should be light and bright.

Use of Colour Patches

This is by far the most popular and inexpensive means of utilising colour therapy. Small square-shaped patches of varying sizes can be made from different coloured cloths. Varieties of coloured cloths are available in cut-piece stores selling material for making blouses. These are of standard sizes measured in metres.

However, a little care is necessary while buying coloured cloth. Do not buy cloth in the evening or night under artificial light, as the shades look different. Always buy after examining the shade in sunlight. You can use either cotton or silk, as both are easily available. Synthetic materials should not be used.

The size of the cloth you require depends on the area of application. For chakra healing, you need sizes of not more than 3″ × 3″. To enable easy handling make several folds of this size and stitch all round. It then sits properly on the body above the spot to be treated.

All the seven coloured pads can be treated in this manner and used for chakra healing, which is described in a subsequent chapter.

For spot treatment you will need a cloth piece of bigger size. Examine the area where the colour is to be applied and cut the cloth into the required size.

For areas like the arms or legs, you can utilise a sufficient length of cloth that goes all round and then use a cotton band to keep it in place.

For areas like the stomach, it is fine if the size of the cloth is just sufficient to cover the area to be treated.

By stitching cotton tapes at the ends and using a little imagination, it is possible to make treatment pads that stay in place for the desired length of time.

Colour through Interiors

By making appropriate choices, colours can be effectively used to bring health and cheer for everyone in the family and to nurse the sick back to health.

Colours used in furnishings can be changed to healing colour shades in the patient's room, especially those of chronic ones. This will not only result in speedy healing, but also make the patient more optimistic, cheerful and energetic, resulting in faster recovery.

A colour should always match the other colours present in a room. For example, if you are using a particular shade of carpet in the room, that colour should go well with the colours of the curtain, walls, etc.

Painting of Walls

The other way of introducing colours is by painting the walls in the desired colour. Before painting, choose the colour carefully and be sure that the colour is to your liking and is the one needed under the circumstances.

Painting of walls is ideal when the complaint is chronic and treatment for a long period is required. This method can be chosen when only one colour is recommended for healing.

It is always better to first use materials of that colour like bedspreads, curtains, blinds, etc. Once you are sure that this colour suits the patient, you can go in for that colour.

To have the benefit of colour for all family members, use those colours that are energising and agreeable to all. Normally, sky blue, white and green are nature's colours and use of these colours has beneficial effects.

Colour Treatment through Water

When water is exposed to sunlight, it gets energised. This type of water energising is called *solarising*. Sunlight contains seven colours and each colour has its own effect on various organs of the body. It is possible to prepare specific coloured solarised water by using coloured glass. As it is difficult to get specific coloured glasses, the normal method is to take a colourless glass bottle and wrap it with transparent paper of the desired colour.

Depending upon the colour that is used to solarise the water, it is referred to as 'red solarised', 'blue solarised', etc. The amount of time required for this depends upon the season. In summer, charging is quick, whereas in winter, the charging is slow. Exposing water to sunlight for ten minutes' duration is considered adequate for most purposes.

One can prepare several bottles of solarised water and consume this at regular intervals throughout the day. Water should always be sipped so that the sensitive cells of the tongue absorb the energy.

Once solarised, water can be stored in the refrigerator. However, it is not advisable to store the water for a number of days at a time. The maximum duration allowed by colour therapists is 48 hours after charging. Thereafter, the potency comes down and it may not be advisable to consume such water.

While consuming colour solarised water, refer to the previous chapter, where colours for various illnesses are mentioned. The same chart is to be applied here as well.

Coloured Garments for Good Health

Another method of administering colour therapy is to use the healing colour in body wear. Here again, select the colour that is needed and wear it in the initial stages for a couple of hours. Watch the body's reaction. If it is agreeable, increase the duration till a cure is obtained.

It is often said that the colours we wear reflect our personality. Colours also have the ability to bring out the best or the worst in us. You must have observed that certain people look very active, lively and healthy in some clothes, whereas the same person wearing garments of another colour looks pale and ill.

The way a person appears to you is exactly the way the colour is acting on him. If a person appears lively and healthy in garments of a particular colour, then that is the colour he needs to stay healthy and active. If a person looks pale in garments of another colour, then this is the colour he should avoid, as wearing the wrong colours will eventually make him sick.

Colours Alter Mood

For example, if a person is depressed, he should not use colours like grey, black or faded colours. These can aggravate the situation. The use of bright colours will have a salutary effect on his mind and help him come out of the depression.

Similarly, when a person feels low on confidence, he should use bright colours that attract attention. On the other hand, if one is irritable or under stress, he should use calming colours like light blue, violet, etc. It is not always necessary to use colour in the form of body wear. One can use it with equal effectiveness in bedspreads, pillow covers, curtains etc.

While it may not always be possible to use garments of a desired colour, this problem does not arise when it comes to the question of pillow covers or bedspreads. So, it is always better to make changes here if a particular colour is unsuitable as dress material.

Effects of Specific Colours

Red has a stimulating action on the heart and circulatory system. It helps you feel strong and energetic and is associated with vitality and ambition.

Pink is a mixture of red and white, and has a gentler action than red. It is emotionally soothing and calming. It lessens feelings of irritation, aggression, loneliness and discouragement and helps us feel less burdened and more confident.

Orange strengthens digestion and the immune system. It is a happy colour, easing emotions and boosting self-esteem. It creates enthusiasm for life. Orange mixed with white creates tones of apricot and peach, which are good in moments of emotional exhaustion.

Yellow strengthens the nervous system. It makes one more clear-headed and alert. It is a happy and uplifting colour, allowing clear thinking for decision-making. Yellow helps by changing one's attitude into an optimistic one.

Green helps regulate circulation. It is the colour of the heart, both physically and emotionally. It helps open the heart so we may be more empathetic to those around us.

It is a colour we are often drawn to when under emotional stress, because it promotes relaxation and calmness and soothes emotions.

Blue light has been shown to lower blood pressure, is anti-inflammatory and has pain-relieving properties. Blue is very calming and cooling and associated with a higher part of the brain. It promotes mental control, clear thinking and inspires creative thought. Dark blues help us connect to our intuitive and feminine side.

Purple and **violet** have a purifying, antiseptic effect, and are physically cooling. These colours are also associated with a higher part of the brain, encouraging intuition and feelings of being more connected psychically. They are often worn for psychic protection and are connected with many of our higher senses – sensitivity, spirituality, compassion and higher ideals. Like blue, these colours stimulate creativity and inspiration.

White is the colour of purity, protection and peace. It has a cleansing effect on the emotions and the spirit. It can create space to think, but too much white is too cooling and isolating.

Black is associated with the feminine nature of things, both comforting and protecting. It gives an air of mystery to the wearer. Overuse of black clothes can be too reserved and inhibiting. This can be avoided by mixing it with other colours like gold. Yellow is energising, mentally stimulating and associated with power and abundance, which is beneficial with black.

Brown is a stabilising colour, helping you feel connected to the earth. It helps with being more nurturing and supportive. Too much brown, though, can decrease your feelings of self-worth. Mix it with other colours.

This is only a very brief description of how the major colours affect you physically, emotionally and spiritually.

Colour Therapy through Food

The colour of food is linked to the characteristics of the colour. In the Colour Therapy Chart, if the colour that is recommended cannot be introduced in any other manner, you can get the benefit of colour therapy by just switching over to the recommended colour foods.

If you need red colour to recover from any ailment, then you can use beetroot, watermelon, tomato and strawberry. If your element calls for the use of yellow colour, eat bananas, papaya, the yolk of eggs, etc. If you need blue colour, eat grapes and brinjals. If you need orange colour, have oranges or carrots.

OOO

Colour Breathing Techniques

This is another variation of colour therapy. However, as visualisation is involved, here your active participation will be required. Colour breathing can be practised at any time of the day or night. It can also be practised when one is about to retire to bed or immediately after getting up from bed.

It is mostly practised to maintain good health. However, it can also be practised to cure a disease.

Method: Make sure that you are comfortable and relaxed. Sit on a comfortable chair and rest your legs in a position that you find most relaxing. You can also lie on your back on a mat or cot. Breathe calmly by taking a deep and slow breath. Now imagine that white light is entering your head from outer space and all your organs are filled with this light. Hold this image for two minutes.

Now, think of the colour you like best. Again, imagine that the entire room is filled with this colour and you are bathed in it.

During Sickness

If you have a health problem that requires the use of red, yellow or orange colour, imagine that this particular colour is emerging from the earth, you are standing at its centre point and the colour is engulfing you from feet to the head.

If your ailment calls for the use of blue, violet or indigo, imagine that a coloured beam from the sky of that particular colour is descending on your head and bathing you from head to toe. If, for example, green is the colour recommended in your case, then stand on your feet with arms relaxed, imagine a green beam coming on your head and entering the body. A part of the green light is movin towards your head and another part is moving towards your feet. This colour exercise is to be done for a maximum duration of three to four minutes at a time.

Imagine the colour that is needed for healing and imagine that you are inhaling that colour and it is spreading from the lungs into your entire body. When you breathe out, always imagine that the colour has changed into another complementary colour. For example, if you have inhaled red, the exhalation colour will be yellow. If you have inhaled blue, the exhalation colour will be violet and so on.

At the end of the exercise, again imagine that you are being engulfed by white light and cleansed thoroughly.

One problem in this method is the difficulty experienced by patients with visualisation, which is a technique that needs some practice to master. Not all people are good visualisers. While some can visualise very clear images, others find it difficult to get any image in their mind's eye. This normally happens when people start visualisation techniques for the first time.

However, visualisation can be mastered by anybody with some effort and one need not consider it to be a special gift. In the beginning if it becomes very difficult for you to imagine the colours, the best way to go about it is to first create the colour physically. Bring the appropriate coloured paper and create the coloured light you need by covering a clear bulb with that colour.

Spending some time physically with colour makes it easy for you to visualise these.

Distant Healing

Like Reiki, colour healing is also practised as a distant healing method. Here the healer first identifies the colour that is required to cure the patient. Distances in such cases are not a deterrent, as colour is believed to travel with the speed of light and almost instantaneously the energy reaches the patient.

Once the healer selects the right colour, he makes a beam and imagines that the beam is going from him to the patient. This is as effective as the patient himself being exposed to the colour.

In many a case, where the patient is physically or mentally unable to involve himself in colour therapy, distant healing is the only method by which the benefits of colour therapy can be made available to the patient.

It is not necessary that there should be some distance between the healer and the patient. Anybody in the family can sit in one room and send colour vibrations to a patient lying in the other room. Several colour therapists have reported instantaneous cures, since colour healing is basically healing of the Aura and once the Aura is healed, recovery is almost immediate.

Meditation is an invaluable aid in improving visualisation techniques. When a person sits for meditation, he is usually flooded with numerous thoughts. But as he continues to prune thoughts that arise in his mind, these go on decreasing.

Studies on techniques like transcendental meditation carried out by several universities across the USA have conclusively established that, while thoughts will flood the mind in the initial stages, as one progresses, the number of thoughts go on decreasing till a time is reached when there are hardly any thoughts and the person feels calm and relaxed. It is what Maharshi Mahesh Yogi refers to as 'restful alertness'. The mind is calm when this stage is reached and visualisation becomes easy.

Normally, failure to visualise something is only because there are too many other thoughts crowding our mind. These thoughts come in the way of visualisation. Once the mind is calm, visualisation becomes effortless and you will be able to visualise the colour you need.

In the initial stages of meditation, even if the eyes are closed, a man hardly feels it is pitch black, although no light is entering. Normally, one sees a greyish blackness, which changes over a course of time to pitch darkness.

If you can see pitch darkness when your eyes are closed, it means your mind is controlled enough to start the visualisation technique.

It is not necessary that you have to follow a system of meditation to arrive at this level. Closing the eyes and doing rhythmic breathing is all that is required to reach this stage over a course of time. Once this stage is reached, you will be able to visualise whichever colour you need.

The same technique can be used to heal others as well. If you can visualise the colour that is required in your mind's eye, you can easily direct that colour to the patient, irrespective of the distance. One advantage of colour healing is that the healer instantaneously senses when the healing is complete. Once the patient absorbs all he can and stages a recovery at the aura level, a healer experiences a reduction in the colour that is drawn from him.

In other words, if the colour sent from him is absorbed slowly or is not absorbed at all, the healer will still know when the therapy is complete.

Colour Combination Treatment

It is sometimes found that a single colour is unable to cure the disease. This is especially true in the case of chronic complaints like asthma and also with complaints that are several years old. In all these cases, a combination of colours has proved to be more effective in bringing faster relief and cure.

Here is a list of cases where combination therapy is recommended.

Arthritis

This is one condition where almost all systems of medicine fail most of the time. Although modern medicine and surgery come to the rescue, the pain associated with this disease and the prohibitive cost of surgical treatment have made every person fear the onslaught of this disease.

Arthritis starts as a pain in the joints and muscles, which radiates to different parts of the body. Slowly, the joint gets affected and it becomes difficult for the patient to even go through day-to-day activities. Much of the treatment is aimed at alleviating the pain but the painkillers prescribed are not without side effects.

Secondly, in the course of time, the body becomes immune to every painkilling drug prescribed, and even higher dosages fail to produce significant results.

This has necessitated the introduction of steroids and more powerful painkilling drugs, which may result in the total collapse of some other organ system. Arthritis responds favourably to colour therapy and most colour therapists have a large clientele of arthritis patients. However, the victims can easily practise colour therapy at home.

For arthritis, three colours have to be used simultaneously – blue, green and orange. Each colour has to be given for at least 50 minutes daily, but blue can be given for a longer duration. The treatment should start with blue colour, as this soothes and relieves pain.

After treating with blue, green colour treatment should be given, as green energises the affected portion of the body. Thereafter, orange colour is required, which makes all cells in the affected area release their toxins and goads them to work efficiently.

It is easy to apply this colour by using coloured bulbs, as blue, green and yellow bulbs are readily available. You can easily use it. The combination of these three colours can also be used in rheumatism, where the pain is more severe.

Lack of Immunity

Proper functioning of the immune system is absolutely essential to maintain perfect health. The increased levels of pollution as well as the quality of air we breathe and the water we drink have all put the immune system under great stress.

The exploding population in urban centres promotes the spread of disease, with airborne and waterborne diseases being very common in urban areas. Immunity is the greatest protection against any contagious disease. If immunity is at its peak, a large number of diseases can be warded off.

An attack of frequent colds, fevers and infection based on gastrointestinal disorders all point to the unsatisfactory functioning of the immune system. Failure of the immune system has a cascading effect and every attack strains the system further, opening the way for another attack. Thereby, a person suffers from endless complaints when the immune system is weak. Antibiotics give only temporary relief.

In all such cases, exposing the person to a combination of orange, green and yellow colour can strengthen the immune system. The treatment should start with orange, followed by green and end with yellow. The minimum period of treatment is 15 minutes with two sessions per day.

This is ideal for children who fall sick frequently.

Diabetes

Diabetes is another disease that responds well to combination colour therapy. Diabetes is the inability of the body to effectively use insulin released by the pancreas, which is required for proper ingestion of foods. There is no cure for diabetes in any other system of medicine, but one can regulate the disease by a combination of exercise, diet and medication.

Combination colour therapy has been found to bring remarkable relief in all cases of diabetes. Located on the left side of the abdominal area, the malfunctioning of the pancreas results in diabetes.

A treatment of 30 minutes with green colour, followed by yellow colour for 15 minutes and red for 10 minutes, makes the gland secrete the right quantity of insulin and strengthens the organ.

Combination Therapy in Psychosomatic Disorders

Psychosomatic disorders are physical ailments that arise due to emotional causes. Modern psychiatry can identify psychosomatic disorders and differentiate these from physical ones.

But the treatment of psychosomatic disorders and the success rate are rather below par. This is because the patient's co-operation is very essential to administer healing effectively, unlike in the case of other physical disorders where the drug alone can bring about a cure.

Combination therapy can bring substantial relief for patients with psychosomatic problems. Three colours are selected for such problems – red, yellow and green. To start with, red is given for 15 minutes, followed by yellow and then green, for 15 minutes each.

Menopause

This is a stressful period for most women. Menopause normally occurs between the age of 40 and 50. A woman undergoing menopause experiences uncomfortable hot flashes and exhibits symptoms of nervousness. They also become irritable and experience a lack of vitality and energy.

A combination therapy of blue, yellow and green can help them get over the problem. The ideal way to take the treatment is to allow the light to fall on the uncovered abdominal area. Begin with blue and follow this up with yellow and green for 10 minutes each.

Gradually, the duration can be increased, depending on the tolerance level of the patient.

Migraine

This is a baffling complaint that does not have any satisfactory medication. Migraine sufferers experience painful headaches for long durations. The causes of migraine are still not clearly known, although it is believed these are psychosomatic in nature.

The combination of colours used to treat migraine are red, yellow, blue and green. Red is first used to boost circulation, followed by yellow, which clears the liver of toxins. Then comes blue, which is a cooling and soothing colour. The session ends with green, which is nature's healing colour and heals both at the mental level and physical level.

In addition to this, a patient can also use beetroot to stimulate the benefits of red colour, banana for the benefits of yellow colour, green vegetables to stimulate the healing of green and grapes to get the benefits of blue.

In case of severe migraine, the morning session can consist of red, blue, green and yellow, while the evening session may consist of 15 minutes of colour therapy with only blue and violet colours. This ensures good sleep, which helps the person cope with disease in a better frame of mind.

Obesity

This is a common complaint of the middle-aged modern man. Lack of physical exercise, eating of high-calorie food and predisposition to the accumulation of fat are some of the factors cited for this disease.

Obesity is now considered a disease in itself, since it can bring on a host of other complaints like blood pressure, diabetes, heart problems and even cancer. Usually, obesity is determined by calculating the body mass index.

BODY MASS INDEX TABLE

Standard Heights and Weights for Men and Women (Medium Frame) (For 25 years and above)

MEN

Height		*Weight (kg.)*
Cms.	*Ft.*	
157	5′2″	56.3-60.3
160	5′3″	57.6-61.7
162	5′4″	58.9-63.5
165	5′5″	60.8-65.3
168	5′6″	62.2-66.7
170	5′7″	64.0-68.5
173	5′8″	65.8-70.8
175	5′9″	67.6-72.6
178	5′10″	69.4-74.4
180	5′11″	71.2-76.2
183	6′0″	73.0-78.5
185	6′1″	75.3-80.7
188	6′2″	77.6-83.5
190	6′3″	79.8-85.9

WOMEN		
Height		Weight (kg.)
Cms.	Ft.	
152	5′0″	50.8-54.4
155	5′1″	51.7-55.3
157	5′2″	53.1-56.7
160	5′3″	54.4-58.1
162	5′4″	56.3-59.9
165	5′5″	57.6-61.2
168	5′6″	58.9-63.5
170	5′7″	60.8-65.3
173	5′8″	62.2-66.7
175	5′9″	64.0-68.5
178	5′10″	65.8-70.3
180	5′11″	67.1-71.7
183	6′0″	68.5-73.9

Once obesity occurs, it is rather difficult to lose excessive weight. The problem with obesity is that the person feels an uncontrollable urge to eat wrong foods, fully aware of the fact that he is obese. Colour therapy basically aims at suppressing the obesity mechanism in the patient.

Once the patient has reduced appetite, the chances of indulgence are very remote. For this, a combination of violet and pink is used. For instance, in your dining area if you use violet colour on the wall and pink-coloured mats on the dining table and pink-coloured light in the room, your appetite will diminish and you will be satisfied with a few spoonfuls of food.

John Hopkins Medical University in Baltimore conducted a study where patients were asked to wear a pink-coloured square-shaped cloth. They found that this not only reduced the appetite of patients, but also brought down violent tendencies in oversensitive patients. It also controlled stress-related snacking.

OOO

Colour Therapy Through Chakras

One of the most popular methods of healing is to treat the chakras associated with the ailment and effect a cure.

In a previous chapter, we elaborated upon the various chakras and the organs that come under their influence. In other words, the energy from the chakra is supplied to these organs, which in turn take part in physiological activities.

Any illness has its roots in a faulty chakra. If the chakra is unable to control and supply the necessary pranic energy, the organ becomes weak and a disease surfaces. It is important to recognise that the actual problem is not in the organ but in the chakra and setting right the energy imbalance in the chakra can result in the organ regaining its health.

The same colour pads you have made for spot treatment can be used here. Different colour pads of at least 4 x 4 inches are required to cover the mouth of the chakra. Keep the required colour on the affected chakra to secure relief.

Energising Technique for Good Health

Even if a person is healthy, as a preventive measure one should charge the chakras with the appropriate colour. Any illness basically starts with a chakra, which goes out of balance before this manifests itself in the body as an ailment. The best way to charge the chakras is to make a band two inches wide with colour patches of all seven colours at appropriate distances.

Of course, this means more than one user can use a band. But as it is inexpensive, each member of the household can get a band made to suit his height. A person can lie down and place the band in such a way that the appropriate colours are transmitted to the area of a particular chakra.

This way, every chakra absorbs the required colour and remains at the appropriate energy levels. Each band is of the size 2″ x 2″ size. The bands are made in the following colours: violet, indigo, blue, green, yellow, orange and red.

Band Chart

The ideal way to make colour bands is to paint these colours on the band. Then lie down on the floor and keep these cards over the appropriate position of the chakras and start deep breathing.

Concentrate your breath on each band imagining its colour. If you have difficulty in visualising the colour, keep an extra set of patches by your side and take out the card of the required colour, open your eyes, look at it for a couple of seconds and then put it back.

Now, you will be able to visualise the colour more clearly. Imagine that the colour is entering the chakra, through a funnel, the chakra is in a conical shape and the pointed end of the cone is attached to your spinal cord.

If you suffer from any ailment that needs a specific colour, the best way to start this exercise is to first concentrate on the specific colour required by the chakra. Take a couple of breaths and work on it, till you get the feeling that the chakra is getting energised.

Do note that the chakras have cool and hot characteristics just like the colours, and the colour you are absorbing will influence your body in a particular manner. For example, if you are absorbing red, you should feel a sensation of heat. If you are absorbing blue, you should feel a cool sensation sweeping through your body. Once you get this feeling, you can be sure that the colour energy has reached the chakra in the right level.

After doing this exercise, you can switch over to full chakra breathing by taking 10 breaths for each colour, starting from your head to the end of the spinal column.

This not only strengthens and harmonises all the chakras, but keeps you away from all debilitating diseases.

Once you get the feeling that you are completely charged, you can remove the band and keep this for the next session.

OOO

Acupuncture and LED Light Colour Therapy

Acupuncture is of Chinese origin. The system is divided into two parts. One is called Ocular Acupuncture and the other is termed Whole Body Acupuncture.

Ocular acupuncture is based on the principle that an area in the outer ear represents every organ in the human body and stimulating the ear connected with the organ can effect a cure. Several acupuncturists practise ocular acupuncture exclusively. Special acupuncture machines are also used to give mild electrical impulses to various points of the outer ear.

Especially popular has been the ocular acupuncture method to treat high blood pressure, which was also accorded approval by the US Food and Drug Administration as an effective non-drug therapy for controlling high blood pressure.

Where whole body acupuncture is concerned, the principle is different. According to this system, *chi* (cosmic energy or *prana*) flows through special channels called meridians, which are distributed from head to toe. Sometimes these are found just below the skin, while the same meridian is buried deep under the skin in other areas. The point at which it is easily accessible is usually the point where the treatment is given.

According to acupuncture, any illness is basically due to obstruction of the life force or *chi*. The acupuncturist first locates the meridian carrying the life force to the diseased organ. He then cleans the block by inserting needles. This method of clearing blocks by the application of needles is an age-old method of treatment.

However, as technology advanced, the method of treatment also changed. While the basic principle of treating diseases through the meridian channel is still respected, the modern acupuncturist uses special hand-held electrical stimulators, which not only locate the meridian but also pass on electrical impulses to them.

This is one method that is more or less a self-help method where one need not hire the services of a doctor, as there are virtually no contraindications on using such therapeutic tools. These machines are sold in plenty all over the world.

However, the amount of stimulation at any particular point with the use of these machines is rather mild and it may take considerable amount of time before the relief is felt.

Colour Therapy Interpretation in Acupuncture

Acupuncture believes that colour can affect the body's meridians and in the book, *The Book of Knowledge: The Keys of Enoch*, published in 1973, Dr James J. Hurtak established the fact that coloured lights applied to various areas of the body brought changes in the functioning of an organism.

There was a time when even various coloured glasses were prescribed to cure different diseases based on the theory that the retina rods are linked to neurotransmitters, which in turn control pituitary gland and pineal gland functions. Sunlight therapy was probably the most popular and the earliest form of therapy, which uses the meridians to bring about a cure, according to acupuncturists.

Monochromatic Light in Acupuncture

Monochromatic light is a light obtained from an electrical bulb that contains only one frequency. A concentrated beam of monochromatic light acts more like a needle and can be used in the same way as needles are used in acupuncture.

One advantage with monochromatic light (MRLT therapy) is that unlike needles that are passive, monochromatic red light therapy supplies an abundant amount of concentrated form of force to the required meridian, which aids very fast recovery.

In fact, MRLT is the only method where substantial relief has been obtained in cases of migraine, which defies all other functional forms of therapies. Similarly, asthma and arthritis – which do not yield easily to conventional therapeutic methods – give very good results when treated with MRLT.

The advantage of MRLT is that it can also be applied directly to the point where the pain is felt and even a five-minute application directly to the point of pain gives substantial relief. Hence, it can be used both to treat acupuncture points as well as for spot treatment.

Monochromatic light can be derived from two sources:

1. Soft laser
2. LED lights

Soft laser therapy is popular in the West but only qualified therapists can give it, since overexposure can lead to side effects.

LED (Light-emitting Diode) lights are safer. Today LED lights are available up to 8,000 mini-lumen brightness. The ones you see on electronic equipment are only 15 mini-lumen. The only difference between LED and laser is that although both produce monochromatic light, the light from LED is not coherent, whereas the laser beam is coherent.

According to therapists, though, this factor does not matter, since the cells respond as long as the light is monochromatic. LED therapy is free from side effects and safe. It can be given as spot treatment or on acupuncture points.

As these treatments are free from side effects, anyone in need of relief can undertake this therapy. However, this therapy is best given by a qualified acupuncturist. When this is not possible, a patient can use the acupuncture charts available at most homeopathic outlets (these are also available on various websites) and resort to self-treatment.

Energy Colour Healing

So far we have spoken about how to use the vibration energy of colours for curing various ailments. Recent advances in colour therapy have discovered ways of combining vibration energy of colours with the bio-energy medium and delivering it to the body. This is a far more effective method, as any imbalance in the body's bio-energy field is also automatically corrected.

According to the holistic method of treatment, bio-energy stands at the base of health and disease. If there is sufficient bio-energy in the body, a person will have good immunity and enjoy good health. If the bio-energy level falls, the immunity comes down and he will either be prone to infections or to other chronic diseases that may arise from unsatisfactory functioning of various organ systems in the body.

There are several systems based on this principle like pranic healing, Reiki, energy healing and so on. Pyramids have been known from time immemorial as energy devices. The word 'pyramid' comes from the Greek, *pyra* (fire) and *mid* (middle or centre). In other words, the word pyramid stands for fire or energy at the centre.

A pyramid creates an energy field inside, which studies have confirmed is nothing but a condensed form of pranic energy. The energy is released in the pyramid at about one-third the height on the centre line joining the apex and the point of the base.

Pyramids have become popular energy devices all over the world. These come in various sizes and even man-sized pyramids are available for meditating as well as sleeping.

Pyramids are normally made in the proportion of the Giza Pyramid of Egypt. Here there is a close relation between the base and the sides of the pyramid. Slight variations in the dimensions of the pyramid do not seem to affect the power of the pyramid.

The following dimensions have been found to be quite suitable. Base 9.5″, side 9.00″ and centre height 9.00″. Another type of pyramid with a somewhat varied dimension is also popular: Base 10.5″, side 10″ and height 7″ (approximate).

In practice, both pyramids are found to be quite effective. These sizes are ideal for use in colour pyramid therapy.

Pyramid Material

Pyramids can be made from various materials. Although cardboard pyramids can be easily fabricated, they are not very suitable for long-term use, since cardboard lacks the necessary rigidity and ease of handling. Because of these problems, cardboard pyramids are unsuitable for healing purposes.

Plywood pyramids are available in the market, but experiments have shown that there is a relationship between the density of the material used and the energy that is generated inside. As plywood is a low-density material, these pyramids are quite weak and are therefore not very suitable for healing purposes.

The best material is fibreglass. Dr Wilhelm Reich, a German scientist who discovered orgone energy (another name for bio-energy), showed that when inorganic material is layered with organic material, bio-energy gets liberated. He kept layers of steel wool and cotton over wooden boxes and successfully cured several ailments by making people spend some time in these boxes.

In fibreglass pyramids, two materials are used. One is polyester resin, an organic material, and the other is glass fibre, which is inorganic. Thus fibreglass sheet is a natural blend of organic layer and creates a more powerful field inside. In addition, fibreglass is rigid, mechanically strong, easy to clean and long-lasting.

In view of the natural advantage that fibreglass enjoys, it is the best choice for pyramids.

Size of the Pyramids

Any power equipment has a relationship to size. Naturally, as the size goes up, the power rating also increases. It is the same with a motor, generator or any other mechanical or electrical equipment.

When it comes to the pyramid, the same analogy applies. Although small pyramids of three or four inches produce power, they fall short of human organism energy levels and are not effective. Experiments show that a minimum size of nine inches is required to create sufficient power if the body is to benefit.

Hence, I would strongly recommend the use of a 9.5-inch standard pyramid or the 10.5-inch epsilon pyramid made out of fibreglass.

As a holistic therapeutic tool, it is advisable to have a set of pyramids that are finished in different colours. Usually, fibreglass pyramids are white. By using standard enamel paints one can have colour pyramids, one each in red, blue, green, yellow, orange, indigo and violet. These types of colour pyramids are used abroad and also sold on websites. Use of these pyramids in place of colour cloth or colour badges is far more effective and the results are much better.

Holistic healers use pyramids as their favourite tool. Two kinds of pyramids are in vogue. One is the man-size pyramids, which are now made in copper tube frame construction, and smaller pyramids with solid faces on all sides. Here, we will discuss solid pyramids only.

Although the pyramid is a healing device by itself, combining it with colours can enhance the healing power of the pyramid. Usually, the three sides are coated with complementary colours so that the chakra can absorb the required colour. Similarly, spot treatment is also given using the same pyramid.

Complementary Colour Pyramids

Making and using complementary colour pyramids can achieve considerable saving. The complementary colours are:

- Red, orange and yellow
- Blue, indigo and violet
- Green, blue and turquoise

In this method, one face is left white to act as a balancer for the energy fields inside and only three faces are coloured. Three such pyramids are adequate for all health problems.

However, an octagonal colour pyramid can replace the use of multiple pyramids in as cost-effective a manner. This is discussed in the next chapter.

ooo

Octagonal Colour Pyramid

There are basically two methods of aligning a four-faced pyramid. These are known as:

1. Face alignment
2. Diagonal alignment

In the case of face alignment, the pyramid is aligned so that each face faces a cardinal direction.

In case of the diagonal alignment, the faces face corner directions and the corner of the pyramid will be facing cardinal directions.

In practice, both the alignments work but depending on various factors, like the deflection of the axis and impact of other electro-magnetic radiations of unknown origin, one alignment appears to work better than the other.

Hence, pyramid users are always advised to try both the alignments and select the one that is more powerful than the other. Superimposing both the alignments, we get the octagonal pyramid.

The octagonal pyramid is therefore a combination of two four-faced pyramids – one aligned on the straight axis and another on the diagonal axis. It combines the power of both pyramids, as all the eight faces are aligned to the respective directions. The pyramid is aligned so that any one face looks at the north. The remaining faces look east, south-east, south, south-west, west and north-west respectively.

This pyramid is very powerful and produces several times more energy than a four-faced pyramid of similar dimensions.

The pyramid can act as a substitute for multiple colour pyramids. The pyramid is made out of fibreglass and has a base of about 11 inches and height of 9 inches. It is generally made in white. Each face is painted with one colour – violet, indigo, blue, green, yellow, orange, turquoise and red.

Keeping the pyramid over the chakras, as described earlier, helps the chakra absorb the required colour. The pyramid is moved over all the chakras and the duration of charging a chakra is maximum three minutes. For the crown chakra one should wear the pyramid as a hat.

For charging the remaining chakras one has to lie flat on one's back and the apex of the pyramid is to be arranged so that it is exactly above the chakra.

Use of Colour Pyramid Water

We have discussed in the earlier chapters how water can be charged with colour energy. Instead of exposing water to coloured lights, you can prepare water charged with the desired colour vibration by using pyramid also. However, here you will need different colour pyramids based on the ailment.

There are two methods of using these pyramids. If the body part is easily accessible to the pranic centre of the pyramid, it is always better to bring the pranic centre of the pyramid close to the affected part.

For example, in case of migraine, the pyramid can be used on top of the head.

Sinus problems: Select the specific colour from the chart given earlier. Lie down on a flat surface. It is always better to lie down north-south, so that the body is in the magnetic axis, and keep the pyramid over your face so that the faces of the pyramid are in line. Now let your body relax in this position for 15 minutes. Note that the apex of the pyramid should be right above the nose.

Tooth problems: Similarly like the above, slide the pyramid so that the apex is above the teeth. For migraine and other headaches, sit on a chair comfortably and wear the pyramid on the head. Here, adjust the alignment of the pyramid so that the four faces are looking at four directions.

Ear problems: For ear problems, lie down on the side and keep it over the affected ear. A similar position is used for ringing in the ear and tinnitus.

Chest problems: For problems connected with chest, use the position as shown in the photograph. Please note that this treatment should be undertaken after ruling out any problems connected with the heart. It is important in all cases of pain in the chest region to rule out any heart or lung problems.

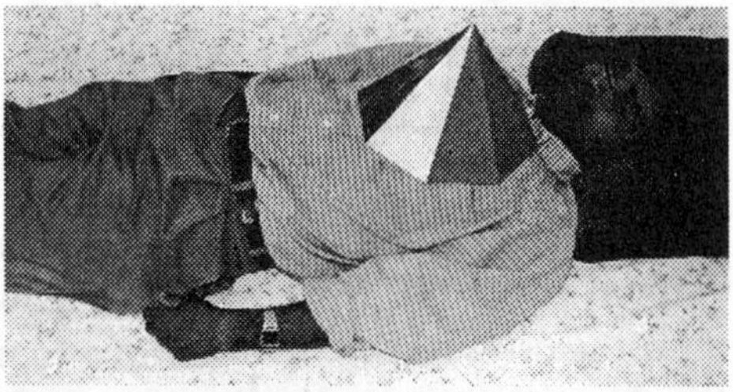

Charging the heart chakra with the octagonal pyramid.

Only when it is ascertained that the pain is due to strained muscles or rib bone, which is normal in middle age, you can use the colour pyramid as complementary therapy along with the medication prescribed by your doctor.

Backache: This is common in middle age and a majority of people suffer from it. The common causes of this problem are lack of exercise, wrong posture while sitting or standing and obesity. It mostly affects sedentary workers.

Before adopting the pyramid treatment, rule out the possibility of slip disc or any other complication, by having a check-up from a qualified orthopaedic surgeon.

When the cause is identified as simple backache and no prolapsed discs are involved, use the therapy with a pyramid. Lie down on your stomach on the north-south axis and ask one of your friends or relatives to place a pyramid on your back so that it comes over the spot where the intensity of pain is the most. Maintain this position for 12 to 15 minutes.

For pain in the legs, sit on a chair and keep your legs on either side and place the pyramid on the area of pain, taking due care to see that the leg does not rest on the floor.

In case of acute sleeping disorders, keep the colour pyramid over the head by making use of it as shown in the figure. The different figures show how to make use of the colour pyramid for various diseases. ooo

Pyramid Healing Through Chakras

The chakra treatment can be given more effectively with the same octagonal pyramid. Start with the crown chakra. For treatment on the crown chakra, you have to necessarily sit in a squatting position or vertically on a chair.

It is recommended that not more than five minutes be spent while charging the chakra with the pyramid energy. After charging the crown chakra, lie down on your back on a hard surface like a carpet.

Now take the octagonal pyramid and keep it over the brow chakra located between the eyebrows. Thereafter, treat the third chakra again with the colour pyramid.

One advantage with energy healing is that there is an inherent intelligence and communication between the body's *prana* and pyramid energy. The body knows the kind of colour vibration required and absorbs only that which is required. The body works on need-based principles and absorbs only the energy required. Even if treatment is carried on for long periods, the absorption will not increase.

Similarly, although the octagonal pyramid contains all the colours and releases the colour vibration of all colours, the chakra is tuned to receive only one colour vibration depending on its placement. Hence, only that colour which pertains to the chakra is absorbed and the rest are rejected.

Here the body acts like a vessel that can only be filled to its capacity. Hence, when a pyramid of two colours is kept on the third chakra and the upper chakra, only the desired colour is drawn by the respective chakra.

Next, keep the pyramid over the heart chakra, which ensures growth, harmony, love and balance. Violet colour can heal the soul and make the person calm. Brow chakra increases intuitive wisdom. Throat chakra improves communication ability.

The third chakra is a solar plexus chakra and the colour vibration required here is yellow.

The solar plexus is believed to be about one inch above the navel. Keep the pyramid over this area for a couple of minutes so that the chakra can absorb energy. This results in clear thinking, confidence and learning.

The second chakra is called the spleen chakra and its colour is orange. Keep the octagonal pyramid over this area for a while. Proper functioning of this chakra gives you creative energy and confidence.

Base chakras are located at the end of the spinal column. Here, the colour vibration needed is red, which stands for strength and individuality. It is seen that red vibrations given from an octagonal pyramid kept in this area can completely cure impotence in a couple of days.

The chakra charging can be undertaken as a means to cure the sick as well as for maintaining good health. You can start with one minute each and slowly increase the time to five minutes at a time. One session per day is more than adequate. Longer durations can be considered in those areas where there is a health problem.

Coloured pyramids have one particular advantage. They can intensify the vibration energy of the colour by combining with pyramid energy.

Even when the pyramid is used to cure an ailment, charge all the chakras for a minute each and then give five minutes' pyramid energy for the chakra related with the disease.

For readers who are interested in trying this themselves, octagonal colour pyramids and four-sided colour pyramids can be obtained from *Suma Traders* in Bangalore at: *91, Givindappa Road, Bangalore – 4.*

ooo

Colour Crystal Cards

One advantage with technological development is that the idea developed for a specific use will find application in other fields. Crystals have been known from time immemorial as energy devices. They have been used in various cultures for improving the environment, keeping away evil forces and for cleansing purposes.

Crystals do have special properties that are unlike any other known material. When they are under mechanical pressure, they produce a small quantity of electricity. When the electrical field is applied, they show signs of mechanical stress. These properties have been used in the modern world to make electronic watches.

Oscillators are one of the primary components in all telecommunication devices. These modern telecommunication equipments heavily rely on this special property of the crystal.

When American astronauts entered a spacecraft, they experienced a drain of energy and psychological stress. Scientists surmised that some component of the earth's gravitational field that was lacking in space was responsible for this problem.

Several experiments were conducted to reduce what was thought to be a component of the earth's energy field. When crystals were placed in some small containers in the spacecrafts, the problem appeared to come under control.

Further research showed that pyramid-shaped crystals had a better effect than ordinary ones. The crystals were charged with the earth's mechanical vibration, which is 7.83 Hz. When these crystals were placed in close contact with the body, the astronauts were able to spend a considerable amount of time outside the earth's field without any physical or psychological stress.

Keeping in mind space constraints inside the spacecraft, further improvements were made by NASA. NASA designed crystals made from aluminium and thousands of microscopic pyramid-shaped aluminium cast crystals were etched into the card by a highly complex electromechanical process. These cards essentially carry millions of naturally occurring crystals and are therefore a concentrated form of pyramid energy. After etching, the cards are coated with specific colours, which increase the colour vibrations of a specific colour.

Experiments show that these cards emit negative ions, which are very important for well-being. The area that surrounds us contains positive and negative ions. Most of the test particles carry a positive charge and are therefore considered positive ions. Similarly, positive ions get liberated in plenty due to automobile smoke and other pollution-causing activities.

However, when positive ions are in excess in an environment, they create various health problems, the most common being allergy and asthma. Psychologically, this affects the mood of a person. A person feels depressed, ill at ease and seems to age faster.

On the other hand, an increase in the concentration of negative ions elevates our mood and increases immunity. Plenty of negative ions are released near waterfalls. It is the release of these negative ions that perk up your mood, increase your appetite and make you feel energetic.

The effects of using these cards are similar. The size of credit cards, these cards come in all the basic colours like VIBGYOR (the colours of the spectrum).

Most illnesses of the industrialised world are the result of excessive exposure to various types of harmful energy and waves from television, fluorescent lights, microwave ovens, electronic office equipments, photocopier machines and electrical power lines.

Pollution caused by excessive emission from vehicles has distorted and affected energy waves, which once pampered us all the time. Many scientists are of the view that most chronic ailments are due to the impact of these harmful waves.

Micro-crystal colour cards interact with the person's natural energy and succeed in creating natural harmonic balancing energy. These cards are normally carried on the body. It is imperative that these touch some part of the body. The ideal way is to wear these like a locket, always in touch with the body.

One advantage of micro-crystal products is that these are always made of negative ions and, therefore, an individual does not feel the negative effects of a polluted atmosphere.

NASA reported numerous benefits, including an improvement in day-to-day performance and increased decision-making capacity. There is also a specific reason for selecting aluminium oxide crystal. The chemical composition of the ruby, sapphire and Alexandria gemstones, as far as the crystalline structure is concerned, is akin to aluminium crystals. This is the reason why aluminium crystals are closer to the characteristics of gemstones.

That is why, aluminium oxide crystal is the only metal oxide that is also a gemstone and its crystalline structure employs energy of specific colour vibrations for beneficial effects. It can be worn for any length of time without any adverse effects. As stated earlier, the body is governed by an inherent intelligence mechanism and absorbs only the quantity that it needs, with the rest being automatically rejected.

According to Micro Crystal Products, USA, manufacturers of micro-crystal cards, all users have reported a feeling of balance under all conditions. Kirlian photographs of a person's energy felt before and after using the micro-crystal card show manifold amplification of the body's energy field. Micro-crystal cards are, therefore, the modern method of healing through colour vibrations.

The cards are available in several colours and are also used to cure various ailments by keeping them on the related acupuncture points.

The cards are available in India too and can be purchased online from www.indiainfo.com.

Card Maintenance and Benefits

Kept carefully, the cards are believed to last indefinitely. However, once a week the cards should be washed in running tap water for five minutes.

The benefits of using the card are that it interacts with the person's natural energy. It functions with the person's natural body elements. It is made up of non-toxic natural elements and is safe to use. It may be mentioned here that while some health authorities consider aluminium risky, aluminium oxide crystals are free from this problem.

A micro-crystal card is a naturally negative ion generator. Many people in the US have reported various benefits.

All in all, there is no doubt that as colour therapy comes of age, more people across the globe will discover its wonderful healing benefits... that are natural and safe.

OOO

The Acupressure Handbook

(The Shiatsu Technique)

—Shizuko Yamamoto

&

Patrick McCarty

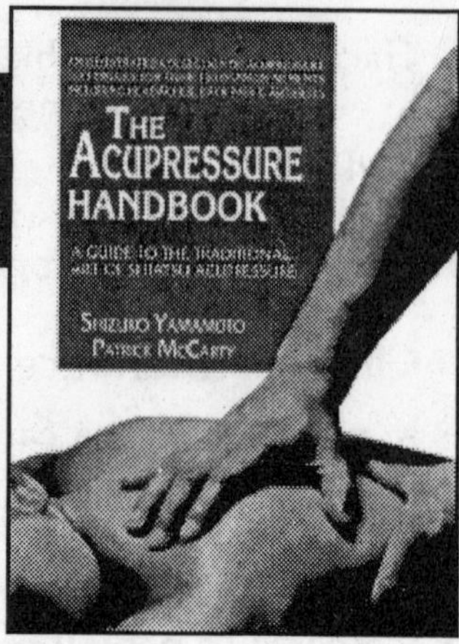

'This unique book is a comprehensive collection of acupressure techniques and natural healing remedies designed to bring about immediate relief from a variety of pains and illnesses. Using easy-to-follow instructions and numerous photographs and illustrations, this book guides you through the various applications of shiatsu massage.

This book is divided into three sections. **Section I,** Foundation, provides a history of shiatsu along with that of macrobiotics. It examines the root causes of illness as well as fundamental principles of the natural forces that affect us all. It shows you how you can draw upon the healing process within each of us. **Section II,** explains how to give a complete shiatsu-acupressure treatment—including the loosening phase, designed to increase circulation and relax the body, and the whole body phase, the pressing and massaging of the neck, shoulders, back, abdomen and arms. A discussion of the various touching techniques is also included. **Section III,** shows you specific acupressure techniques for over 150 common ailments, including allergies, arthritis, asthma, colds, fatigue, hay fever, headaches, high blood pressure, sciatica and more. Throughout the book, the authors provide insights, advice, and practical tips based upon their own years of experience.

Big size, Pages: 264

Price: Rs. 120/- • Postage: Rs. 25/-

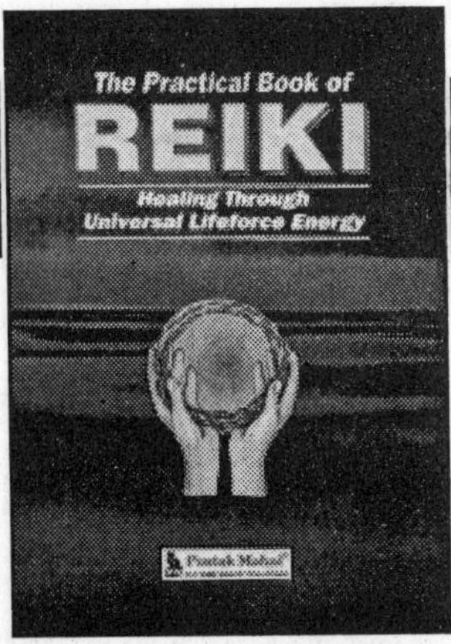

The Practical Book of REIKI

—Mrs. Rashmi Sharma &
Maharaj Krishan Sharma

Healing Through Universal Lifeforce Energy

Find balance and harmony in the mind and spirit. It is truely a gift to yourself!

Increase your vibratory level and healing capacity by treating yourself and others.

Be sure to engage your intuitive knowledge, feel free so that you can maintain the accelerated ability to channel the Reiki energy.

Remove the energy blocks and negative thoughts from Chakras and personality traits.

Apply Reiki by following the five principles:

- Just for today I will live with attitude of gratitude
- Just for today I will not worry
- Just for today I will not anger
- Just for today I will do my work honestly
- Just for today I will show love and respect for every living thing.

This unique book is for those who are looking for a useful treatise for self-treatment and transformation with the principles of Reiki. It is a practical guide that tells you in a plain language to learn and practice Reiki — the Divine Universal Lifeforce Energy.

Spend your day casual in a series of moment-to-victories!

Big Size • Pages: 168
Price: Rs. 88/- • Postage: Rs. 15/-

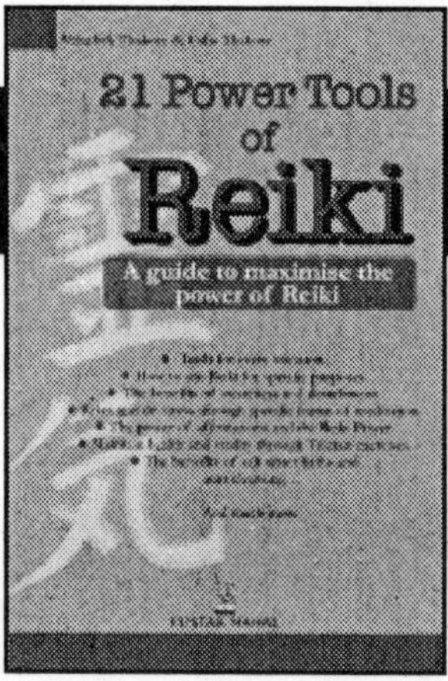

21 Power Tools of Reiki

—Abhishek Thakore
& Usha Thakore

A guide to maximise the power of Reiki

The leading New Age therapy, although extremely popular, Reiki is generally taught at the very basic level. It can, however, do much more than simply heal diseases. Channelled properly, Reiki can be used for very specific purposes with astonishing results. Through the 21 power tools, this book teaches you just how, in a step-by-step manner.

The outcome of five years' research, 21 Power Tools of Reiki is a collection of different methods and tools that make Reiki most effective by concentrating the flow of energy. The book outlines these 21 power tools that you could use for every occasion. Use these tools – and feel the difference!

This book includes: ❖ Tools for every occasion ❖ How to use Reiki for specific purpose ❖ The benefits of awareness and detachment ❖ Relax and de-stress through specific forms of meditation ❖ The power of affirmations and the Reiki Prayer ❖ Maintain health and vitality through Tibetan exercises ❖ The benefits of salt-water baths and aura cleansing…

And much more!

Demy Size • Pages: 136

Price: Rs. 60/- • Postage: Rs. 10/-

AURAS
See Them in Only 60 Seconds!

—Mark Smith

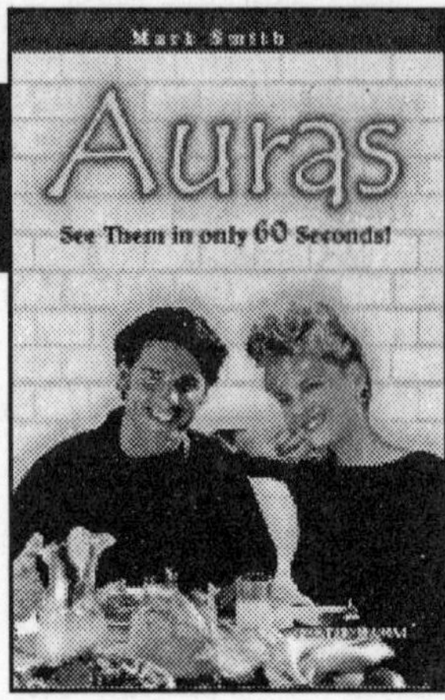

Master the Skill of Seeing Auras!

Your aura is a physical manifestation of your soul, and now you can learn how to see auras for yourself by following ten easy steps. There's nothing metaphysical involved, just simple physics and normal eyesight. Seeing the aura is easy, and Mark Smith shows you how to do it in only 60 seconds!

Learn how the colors of your aura relate to the organs of your body, the chakras, and personality traits. Discover the auric secrets of luminaries and others. Jumpstart your health and well-being through stimulating the energy of your aura with breathing, meditation, and prayer. Alleviate insomnia, stomachaches, and minor pains by simply working with the effects of color on your aura. *Auras: See Them in Only 60 Seconds!* is the ultimate introduction to the emerging spiritual insights to be found within yourself.

Demy Size • Pages: 112
Price: Rs. 60/- • Postage: Rs. 15/-

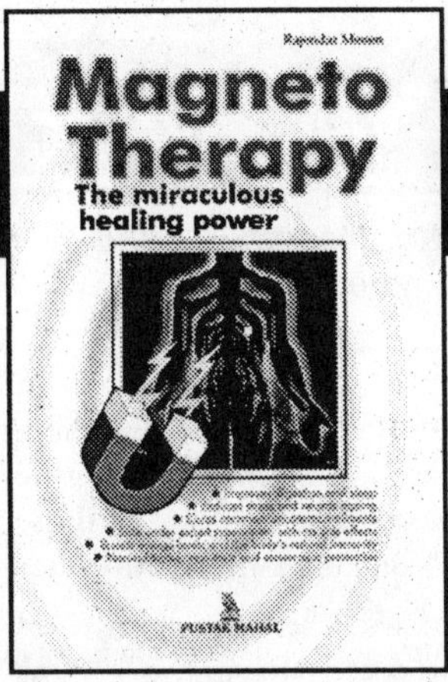

Magneto-Therapy

The miraculous healing power

—Rajendar Menen

Be it an ailment that has you at your wits' end or the fact that you simply seek to enhance your general well-being without burning a hole in your pocket or suffering unforeseen side effects, magneto-therapy is just the right choice for you.

The book is divided into two sections. Section I focuses on magnets, magnetism and magneto-therapy in general and its status in India, while Section II deals with the scenario in the West regarding research, treatments and advances in magneto-therapy. From the origins of magneto-therapy to its current status, from everyday cures to the larger influence of magnets on our lives, from products that are easily available to experiments conducted with magnets all over the world on human, plant and animal life, you will find all this and much more in the book.

If practised properly and diligently, before long you should be eating well, sleeping well and feeling a general sense of well-being at all times.

Demy Size • Pages: 128

Price: Rs. 68/- • Postage: Rs. 15/-

By the Same Author

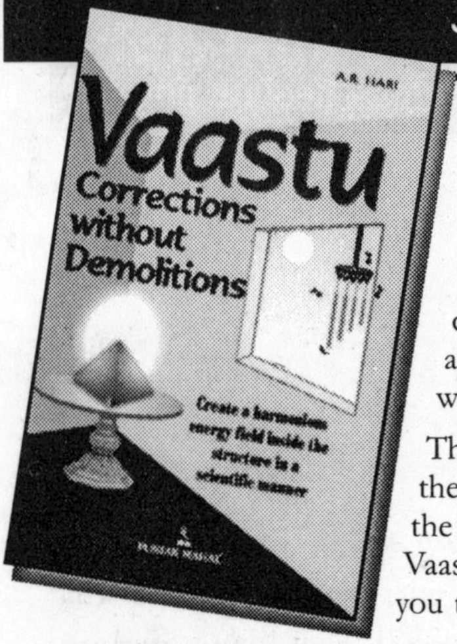

Ensure Health, Happiness and Harmony in Your Home

This book deals with the problem of correcting defective vaastu field where conventional correction methods cannot be applied. This aspect mainly applies to those who live in rented buildings or apartments.

There can also be cases, where the strength of the building and the cost factor may not allow the use of conventional correction methods. Vaastu Corrections without Demolitions helps you to correct Vaastu defects with the help of:

- Feng Shui gadgets
- Installation of Pyramids, Crystals and Ionisers etc.

Demy Size • Pages: 92 • Price: Rs. 48/- • Postage: Rs. 10/-

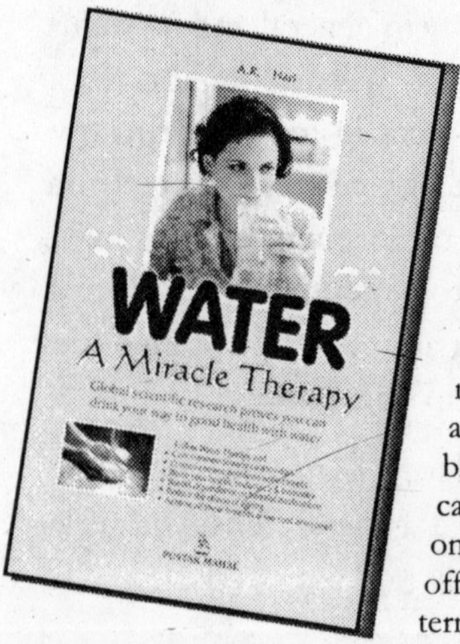

The more science has advanced, the further away have we moved from Mother Nature. Thanks to our artificial existence, even to quench a natural urge like thirst, we imbibe synthetic substances such as coals and caffeine-loaded drinks.

Having starved our body of Nature's most precious liquid, water, we are beset with multiple ailments like headaches, arthritis, asthma, urinary problems, general debility, blood pressure and the like. Missing the root cause of the problem, we rush to doctors—only to have antibiotics pumped into us that offer short-term "relief" while turning into long-term nightmares.

This book shows how drinking just 12 to 14 glasses of water per day (for the average person) cures many ailments, including chronic ones. Incredibly, by just carefully following the Water Protocol in the book, you may feel the difference within 48 hours! Just like a water-starved house plant that springs to attention within minutes of being watered.

Demy Size • Pages: 112 • Price: Rs. 60/- • Postage: Rs. 15/-